- the categons (r&a) have been directive
- Latino, reacting to this directive? trying to reformulate it w/ ethnicity as good

Medicalizing Ethnicity

THE CONSTRUCTION OF LATINO
IDENTITY IN A PSYCHIATRIC SETTING

Vilma Santiago-Irizarry

both rationalize
both fall prey to this issue

- Latino start to themselves as deracing

- Cultural attributes get applied to race

Cornell University Press

Ithaca and London

- Recognize some as doing this concurrently

THIS BOOK HAS BEEN PUBLISHED WITH THE AID OF A GRANT FROM THE HULL
MEMORIAL PUBLICATION FUND OF CORNELL UNIVERSITY.

Portions of this book were adapted from the article "Culture as Cure,"
published in *Cultural Anthropology* 11(1): 3–24 (1996).

First published 2001 by Cornell University Press
First printing, Cornell Paperbacks, 2001

Printed in the United States of America

Library of Congress Cataloging-in-Publication Data
Santiago-Irizarry, Vilma.
   Medicalizing ethnicity : the construction of Latino identity in a
psychiatric setting / Vilma Santiago-Irizarry.
      p. cm.
   Includes bibliographical references and index.
   ISBN 0-8014-3821-7 (cloth)—ISBN 0-8014-8752-8 (pbk.)
   1. Hispanic Americans—Mental health services—New York (State)—New York (City)
2. Psychiatry, Transcultural—New York (State)—New York (City)   3. Ethnopsychology—
New York (State)—New York (City)   I. Title.
   RC451.5.H57 S26 2001
   362.2'089'6807471—dc21   2001001240

Cloth printing   10   9   8   7   6   5   4   3   2   1

Paperback printing   10   9   8   7   6   5   4   3   2   1

For my parents
Felipe Santiago-Díaz
and
Rosa H. Irizarry-Montalvo

It was perhaps also true that those
of us who did not have our origins in the
countries of the mighty West, or North,
had something in common—not, certainly,
anything as simplistic as a unified
"third world" outlook, but at least some
knowledge of what weakness was like, some
awareness of the view from the bottom,
looking up at the descending heel. . . . I
mention this to declare an interest. . . .
I did not go as a wholly neutral observer.
I was not a blank slate.

SALMAN RUSHDIE
The Jaguar's Smile (1987)

Contents

Acknowledgments

In this book I have distilled an enormous amount of diverse data and analysis to focus on ethnicity. I examine, in the specific context of Latino psychiatric care programs, the same cultural principles that I see in my personal and professional experiences in the United States:

Ethnicity is a component of personal and sociocultural identity;
It is unavoidable, and will be imputed by others even when it is not claimed by those who are so labeled;
Society at large variously rewards and penalizes such claims;
One's social persona is often reduced simply to one's ethnic identity.

While I do not wish to condemn the widespread efforts expended on cultural sensitivity, I do advocate for greater understanding of what such efforts mean and the unintended consequences they may bear. I also wish to note that my use of "ethnicity"—as opposed to "race"—follows a logic that I discuss in chapter 1. I am conscious of the debates surrounding the selection and application of either term regarding Latinos in the United States and made my choice on grounds that I found the most productive for this book.

Writing is an individual pursuit; producing knowledge is inescapably a joint venture. It is my privilege to acknowledge the support of a number of collaborators, colleagues, friends, and relatives whose contributions to my work was, and continues to be, crucial to its production. I am, first of all, tremendously indebted to the staff and patients in the Latino programs I

worked with. I hope that I have managed to convey the complexities of the process in which they were so intensely involved.

The research on which this book is based emerged from my participation in an evaluation project, even though my analyses later diverged from the project's initial parameters. This original evaluation was a collective effort, and I am greatly indebted to the research assistants with whom I worked: Anabel Bejarano, Jaime Cárcamo, Steve Edwin, Carmen Polanco, Sally Robles, and Maribel Vargas. Even when informally conveyed and (too often) officially unacknowledged, their critiques of the process of institutionalizing psychiatric programs for Latino patients greatly informed my own.

I am also grateful to my good friend and colleague, Hannah Lessinger, whose sensitive and astute insights so fruitfully uncovered areas of inquiry. Orlando Rodríguez, at Fordham University, was instrumental in the production of this work; his unquestioning support made it possible.

Among the disciplinary gatekeepers who first authorized my entry into anthropology and academia by shepherding me through graduate school and providing me with the ethical orientation and professional standards all teachers and researchers should strive for, I am most grateful to B. B. Schieffelin, Karen Blu, T. O. Beidelman, Fred Myers, and Faye Ginsburg. Davydd Greenwood and Pedro Cabán have helped sustain my faith in anthropology and in a principled and professional academic practice, as have Ana Celia Zentella, Suzanne Oboler, Ted Bestor, and Regna Darnell.

I would not have been able to survive these years without the help of my family, who were understandably puzzled by the prospect of my abandoning an established career, returning to school, and initiating a new career at an age when such changes are often criticized by society. For tactfully withholding judgment, I thank my parents, Felipe Santiago-Díaz and Rosa H. Irizarry-Montalvo, and my sister, Flor Santiago. My only regret is that my mother, who suffers from Alzheimer's, is no longer able to recognize the material tokens of the process—such as this book. I am also beholden to my close friends in Puerto Rico: my fictive and ritual kin, *comadre* and *compadre* Nora Rodríguez-Matías and Raúl Olmo-Olmo and their children, José, Miguel, Pablo, and my *ahijado*, Manuel Olmo. Ángel Hermida and Evelyn Espada and their children, Teresa and Esteban, also graciously suspended their disbelief and consistently demonstrated their utmost support and enthusiasm over these many years. In New York City, my friends Kathleen O'Reilly and Jon Beesing were equally encouraging.

I have been very fortunate in working with a number of brilliant students at New York University, John Jay College, and Cornell University. The dialogues that my students and I have engaged in over the years, in and out of the classroom, have greatly contributed to my own understanding of the institutional processes that I examine. I must acknowledge two students in

particular: Julie Seda-Agrait and Rafael Cox-Alomar. Both Julie and Rafael continue to astound me with their generous intellectual and ideological commitment to helping *nuestra gente* while maintaining a critical perspective that honors the complexity of the Latino condition.

My editor at Cornell University Press, Fran Benson, and series editor Roger Sanjek are to be commended for moving this project along and facilitating its production.

Last (but, of course, proverbially not least), I must acknowledge the support I continue to receive daily from someone I did not even know when I first began working on this book: my husband, Frederic W. Gleach, whose love, intelligence, strength, and integrity have upheld me in multiple ways throughout one of the most difficult periods in my life. At a more tangible level, his critical editing and scholarly suggestions were invaluable.

The data presented came from a study supported in part by grant MH30569 from the Division of Services Research, National Institute of Mental Health, and by contract C-003234 from the New York State Office of Mental Health. The analyses and interpretations are solely mine and by no means reflect the policies and views of these funding agencies.

VILMA SANTIAGO-IRIZARRY

Ithaca, New York

Introduction

This book addresses the medicalization of ethnicity in public mental health care programs in the United States. By "medicalization" I mean the incorporation of ethnicity into medical discourses and practices[1] as a constitutive element of diagnosis and treatment. Ethnicity then becomes an essential—and essentialized—component of a patient's persona that must be isolated, tracked, and addressed by mental health practitioners.

The process I examine here ensued during the implementation of three bilingual, bicultural psychiatric programs for Latino patients in the New York City area.[2] The programs were initiated in the late 1980s through the advocacy of a group of Latino mental health professionals who were explicitly engaged in a political exercise for asserting civic and institutional entitlement. But their proposal also entailed the articulation of "culturally sensitive" modalities of psychiatric assessment and treatment. This dimension became crucial for them, as they believed it could best legitimate the establishment of culturally specific psychiatric programs. Cultural sensitivity required the incorporation of ethnicity, a "soft" categorical entity, into the rational, "hard" realm of medical practice. The institutionalization of the proposed Latino programs thus represented the convergence of political, medical, and institutional interests, not least the revaluation of Latino identity and culture through the production of culturally consonant psychiatric techniques.

These Latino practitioners were attempting to redistribute public health resources and technologies of power for themselves and their patients (Greenwood et al. 1988). This redistribution was not a simple calculation of

costs and benefits, however; "technologies of power" in this context refers
to the ways in which authority is acquired through decisions to implement
specific medical principles, resources, and practices, but it also includes the
morally validating sense of a worthy curative agenda. The Latino project
subsumed goals of personal and collective self-interest in expanding local
labor markets for Latino mental health practitioners and enhancing their
institutional power. Beyond the project's material aspects, however, it also
constituted ideological and symbolic assertions on behalf of "Hispanic people" within the context of a long-standing tradition of communalism, activism, and self-help.

The development of "culturally sensitive" modalities of care, then, was of
utmost importance for these Latino professionals; in their minds, it represented both the project's culminating programmatic goal and its "purest"
animating conceptual principle. Articulating the notion of cultural sensitivity and its insertion into therapeutic techniques reflected their concern with
the relationship between mental illness and culture. It also foregrounded
their desire to reconcile cultural and linguistic difference with the highly rationalized models of care expressed as universalized constructs in psychiatry
and psychology; these constructs inform categories of mental conditions
and behaviors that then become embodied in classificatory grids of diagnosis and treatment. The establishment of these Latino programs validated
the "ethnicization" of mental health care not only as sanctioned public policy, but also, and most important for the Latino professionals involved, also
as rational and enlightened medical practice. The institutionalization of the
programs thus transcended their specific and local nature, manifesting their
potential for wide-ranging medical, political, and symbolic implications for
other ethnic groups.

The purpose of this book is not just to document this process; I argue
here that, ultimately, the worthy leveling agenda espoused by these professionals had the unintended consequences of vitiating their efforts rather
than fully empowering them. Faced with the need for inserting ethnicity
into medical and bureaucratic domains, they found themselves generating
essentialist notions about Latinos and their culture which stressed cultural
and linguistic difference, and thus distance, from the dominant Anglo culture, equally embodied in highly typified terms. Two monolithic, oppositional cultural constructs were thus generated and deployed for the purpose
of validating these programs, erasing the sociocultural and historic specificities of each group as well as the complexities of their history of relations.
Stressing cultural distance paradoxically reinforced the dominant status of
Anglo/Euro-American culture and of the English language as unmarked
categories of identity (Urciuoli 1996).

Equally problematic for me was that, in the attempt to articulate ethnic-

ity with the "medical," "culture" was rendered a reified essence that could be decontextualized from the situated relations that produce it. In practice, the Latino staff in the programs treated elements they deemed "traditional" to Latino culture as concrete referential entities to be identified, isolated, and infused into mainstream psychiatric principles and practices. They eventually reconfigured ethnicity as "content" to the "form" that psychiatric structures, principles, and practices represent, thus subjugating culture to the primacy of medicine—the system into which they had been socialized professionally. I argue that positioning culture in this way contributes to the reproduction of existing conceptual hierarchies that privilege the rationality of medical science over the complex, elusive, and messy construct that is "culture." I also suggest that the broader context for the processes of identity construction that arose in these programs is, ironically, what led to the efforts invested in their implementation: the continuing struggle by Latino groups within the United States to gain access to material and symbolic resources not yet readily available to them, in spite of alleged structural and ideological changes marked by the advent of multiculturalism as the nation's dominant cultural narrative. Multiculturalism in the United States, as I see it, places a premium on cultural difference and rewards its deployment as a controlling argument that validates entitlement.

Of course, the process of identity construction was not as straightforward as I render it here for rhetorical and representational order. It was marked by contradictions and tensions among those involved, causing disjunctures and contestations which I try to convey. I do not mean to argue that these Latino professionals were "unconsciously" deploying these constructs, or that they were all equally blind to the essentializing strategies in which they were engaged. On the contrary, many were conscious of how they were rendering the cultural as an adjunct to the medical or clinical.[3] They were equally cognizant of the structures of inequality through which their own relations to dominant groups in the United States are mediated, as well as of their own authority and elite position vis-à-vis their patients. I have no intention of deprecating their professionalism, decency, and goodwill. Rather, what I am attempting to document are the inherent ambiguities of sociocultural practices. I underscore how the uses of culture, particularly in conditions of structural inequality, are not self-evident, but require an acute consciousness of the unintended outcomes that ensue from the same sociocultural processes that are being mobilized.

The complexities of the situation were (and are) compounded by my own consciousness—shared with others who are members of "problematic" groups in the United States—that it is often necessary to mine dominant sociocultural stereotypes in order to realize empowerment. One's possibilities are understood and rendered viable within the structural conditions and

ideological preferences that prevail in the United States. As noted, this is especially true in these multiculturalist times, when manifestations of ethnicity are ostensibly rewarded by "the system." Rendering identity in essentialist terms—what Wilmsen (1996) terms "primordializing"—then becomes a crucial strategy for advancing political causes among ethno-racial constituencies.

I use the term "medicalizing" deliberately. It underscores one of my main concerns: the power that medical discourses exert upon the processes of ethnicity construction that I examine. I wish to evoke the interaction of mutually articulating categories, processes, and practices—"culture," "the medical," "ethnicity," "identity construction"—within the specific sociocultural domain of medicine and public mental health care. Yet I also wish to stress the ambiguity of these articulations by exploiting the signifying possibilities embodied in the gerund form: "medicalizing." Can ethnic culture be mined and "applied" through therapeutic techniques as the prime curative agent that "medicalizes," that acts as virtual anodyne to repair the social and psychic disjunctures affecting members of groups who live under conditions of cultural and linguistic dissimilarity in the United States? Or, conversely, is ethnic culture the *altering* pathogenic vector that must be subjugated, corrected, and reorganized through therapeutic applications in order to "cure" members of these groups of the effects of a pathologized cultural and linguistic dissonance? The semantic tension lies in the opposition embodied in signifying ethnicity, understood as "culture," as that which "cures" or as that which must be "cured," that which medicalizes or that which must be medicalized. Both aspects, in all their paradoxical nuances and racializing effects, were present in the establishment of the Latino programs I worked with, and both underpin my examination of these programs. The constitutive paradox, as I will show, is rooted in efforts to construe "culture" as at one and the same time pathogenic agent and curative panacea: culture as illness, culture as cure.

In the subsequent chapters I address the construction of local definitions and models of culture, ethnicity, and language. These three elements are structuring processes constructed out of social experience, but that help shape it as well (Geertz 1973:93–94). They are mobilized as forms of knowledge through sets of social practices. Latino professionals and paraprofessionals brought to these programs both explicit and implicit models of ethnic identity, cultural applications, and linguistic ideologies and practices that guided their articulation of the programs' reason for being; but these models were necessarily transformed in the experience. In this case, practical transformations led toward greater typification. Beyond their processual aspects, I take language and culture to be socially constituted systems of cognitive and motivating structures that inform and mediate social interac-

tions (Bourdieu 1977). Ethnicity, in which differentiating parameters of identity are drawn and distinctive significance is assigned to social experience, is operationalized by specifying the collective uniqueness of cultural and linguistic forms, beliefs, and practices. Staff at the Latino programs were invested in the medical culture into which they had been socialized and saw themselves as faced with the task of reconciliating medical discourses and the discourses on ethnicity they were mobilizing. I examine the discursive and practical strategies they developed to accomplish this task, even though their strategies were not necessarily consistent or uncontested.

The issues I address are organized around the ways in which ethnic constructs, as revalued tokens of difference, may enter unexamined into institutional practices and policy making processes and thereby undergo reformulation. The development of culturally sensitive modalities of treatment in the Latino programs was based on constructing ethnicity by essentializing it; once the "essence" of Latino culture had been identified, it could then be isolated, categorized, and treated. At other levels, this aim was articulated as a strategy for legitimating the establishment of the programs. I argue that the programs were also being validated within the domains of medical and bureaucratic ideologies for the presumed "curative" value assigned to their incorporation of "culture"—in the form of ethnic signs and symbols—into the clinical spaces in which they operated.

An underlying issue here is the co-optation of "culture," ethnicity and linguistic ideologies and practices by a hegemonic psychiatric culture. I see this development as an outgrowth of the larger sociocultural context of the United States and equally present in other domains, locally and nationally. The premium placed on a discourse of cultural pluralism in U.S. society opens up domains of practices for the token insertion of ethnicity and the repositioning of subjects within social, political, and economic structures of entitlement. "Native" cultural knowledge is thus eagerly sought and applied to the maintenance of unequal power relations, even while the process produces tangential offshoots that translate into the fragmenting power of resistance.

A general, contemporary co-optation of "culture" in many public domains is used to mark "difference," injecting culture as factor or cause, as an ingredient, discursive and practical, into public and disciplinary analyses. In spite of its focus on culture itself, anthropology occupies an ambiguous position in this trend. It is certainly indexed in other disciplines to validate speculations about the impact of sociocultural factors in whatever field of human activity those fields carve out for themselves. Culture is treated as a matter of common interdisciplinary knowledge, and anthropological notions are applied by scholars and practitioners in other fields to validate the application of a principle of "difference," defined as "problematic" or, pre-

sumably less perversely, as "factor" or "variable" in existing conditions and relationships.

In examining the application of the epidemiological construction of specified populations as "dangerous others," Glick-Schiller has pointed out that

> [e]pidemiologists begin to delineate the factors that put groups of people at high risk for a disease by identifying populations thought to be distinctive along parameters that may increase their degrees of risk. They then begin to search for relationships between factors that characterize each population and the presence or absence of disease among that population. Textbooks in epidemiology carefully specify that a statistical correlation between population characteristics and the presence of a disease does not prove causal relationships. However, the manner in which epidemiologists draw the boundaries to create the population groups is less discussed. (1992:240; citation omitted)

Yet the designation of populations at risk grows out of the larger social context which "shapes decisions about what is considered a risk factor [and] how broadly categories are drawn," and involves "judgment, persuasion, bargaining, and political maneuvering" (Stone, cited in Glick-Schiller 1992:240). Glick-Schiller critiques these effects in the designation of certain populations as being "at risk" for AIDS, whose "culture" is then targeted for the application of "corrective" measures. Here I critique a similar process by which Latinos are generally designated as a population "at risk" for mental illness and thus as prime candidates for the elaboration of culturally sensitive modalities of psychiatric care.

I suggest that anthropologists do not control these applications: as Glick-Schiller (1992:247) goes on to assert, anthropologists draw on the explanatory value of "culture," but it can also be used to obscure relations of domination when it is applied toward framing the experience of certain populations in ways that contribute to the reproduction of their status, particularly in the health field, as "dangerous others." Their behavior is then subjected to analysis directed toward (re)socializing them into presumed "mainstream" norms. I am not negating cultural difference or advocating the dismissal of its effects. But I wish to note that, with the increased application of the concept of culture in policy making, there is an urgent need to gain consciousness of the problematic appropriations it is being subjected to in multiple disciplinary and institutional domains.

Too often, "cultural" knowledge is extracted through a filter of exoticism that perpetuates the differential positioning of those defined as others. The placement of anthropology in the United States as pertaining to the realm of the exotic is thus maintained even while it enters the traffic of other disciplinary discourses. Its liminal disciplinary position potentially renders it

subversive and productive; often, though, anthropology and its practitioners, with differing degrees of consciousness, perpetuate the not so subtle racialization that is recurrent throughout its history and that tarnishes much of past and current disciplinary production.[4] This is evident in many ways large and small; many anthropologists still look askance at studies of the United States. Anthropology's contested role is a topic for other books, however, and beyond my focus here. I note it because it became an overarching concern for me in my efforts to see how the notion of culture was being applied for psychiatric purposes, and because in the encounter with other disciplines and institutional practices that my research has entailed, the experience of having other people's perceptions about anthropology and "culture" reflected back to me has colored my interpretations and shaped my own practice.

The overarching subject of this book is ethnicity, and the people who populate it are self-professed ethnic activists, leaders, and members of elites. But I have tried to place them within the context of the institutional and medical ideologies and practices that informed their actions; their institutional location indexes the larger one of the dominant sociocultural conditions prevalent in the United States. I am "studying up" (Nader 1972): the establishment by Latino professionals of these programs could itself be construed as part of their own process of "moving on up," but it included reaching back to their fellow ethnics. Yet it is not very far to move "up" for these professionals because of the differential positioning that still exists in the United States owing to cultural and linguistic distinctiveness.

This book is not an ethnography as such but an ethnographic study of the paradoxes involved in using notions of culture to validate entitlement in the United States. In chapter 1 I situate the context in which I began to work in the programs and describe how my own interpretations of their establishment transcended the original research agenda that brought me to them. I also address the theoretical constructs of ethnicity that I found most productive in interpreting what occurred in the programs. Last, I describe a series of factors that raised certain methodological issues and shaped my work in the field, as well as its textualization in this book.

Chapter 2 describes the negotiations that led to the establishment of the programs and the actors involved in them. The negotiation process was important because it was there that certain representations about Latinos, Latino culture, and the use by Latinos of the public mental health system converged and were articulated by mental health practitioners, who could claim authority to generate them on the basis of their special occupational and cultural knowledge. These representations shaped the perceptions of Latinos that were incorporated into the proposals, the demonstration projects they generated, and later the programs themselves.

Chapter 3 establishes the local conditions for each of the three programs: their patient populations, organizational structures, clinical spaces, and local histories. Since one of their core programmatic goals was to "ethnicize" the clinical settings in which they were sited, I show how signs of ethnicity were inscribed in the programs' ambiance and in the establishment of "culturally appropriate" activities for their patients, especially as they were held to be consonant with the notion and practice of "milieu" therapy. I argue that these insertions of ethnicity into clinical times and spaces were the strategic product of the programs' political, institutional, and medical goals. That is, Latino staff applied ethnicity toward psychiatric purposes in order to validate the programs as effective bureaucratic creations, ethnic enclaves, and therapeutic exemplars. The ambiguities and paradoxes surrounding this process of ethnicization revolve around the ways in which conditions in the programs challenged the monolithic terms in which "Latino-ness" was being essentialized and objectified in ethnic symbols and signs.

In chapter 4 I address linguistic and cultural ideologies and representations produced locally and applied by program staff. The staff members centered their definitional strategies on two arguments: the first capitalized on demographics, in which Latinos are constituted as important through the magic of numbers; the second involved expectations about a kind of language behavior that amounted, in my mind, to linguistic "regression." These strategies were designed to depict specifically Latino need and to define Latinos in opposition to another major cultural group in New York City, African Americans, as well as to an imagined white "majority." Program staff constructed a Latino "character" quintessentially based on affect. I discuss the paradoxes involved in these strategies, which I characterize as equally empowering and imperfect because the attempt to revalue affect as a constitutive element of Latino culture and character was deployed within various contexts—the United States, clinical settings—that render it of ambiguous and controvertible value. I argue that the focus on affect sustained the therapeutic ideology and clinical practices of the Latino staff, who worked in a medical field in which the affective and the emotional are marked as prime domains for intervention.

Chapter 5 documents the everyday activities that organized institutional life for patients and staff as occasions in which strategies were deployed to fulfill the mandate to develop cultural sensitivity. Staff refracted their own understandings about Latino ethnicity through the terms of psychiatric ideologies and practices. I describe the programs' occupational hierarchies, the categories of assessment and treatment used, and the activities developed in order to establish the immediate institutional context that generated particular kinds of staff-patient interactions. Because psychiatric definitions of

behavior are culturally constructed models for its typification, I argue that staff produced a mode of psychiatric assessment and treatment that appraised Latino attitudes and behavior according to "mainstream" standards reiterated in the psychiatric model—and found Latino ways wanting. They thus rearticulated the overarching characterization of culture as pathogenic even while ostensibly construing it as the prime curative constituent in the programs. Class was a pervasive but unacknowledged ingredient in this process, implicated both in the hierarchical relations between staff and patients and in the occupational hierarchies marking relations between professional and paraprofessional staff.

In my conclusion, I return to the theme of the medicalization of ethnicity. As the institutionalization process evolved in the programs, ethnicity was rendered a psychiatric object of inquiry, assessment, and treatment. I argue that when ethnic behavior and beliefs are thus rearticulated in psychiatric terms, the particular culture or group in question is differentially positioned in terms of notions of "normality" within the dominant society, in spite of the ostensibly empowering agendas that inform the specialized services and programs. Ultimately, though, my account of these processes reiterates Wilmsen's (1996) argument that primordialism is a prevalent subtext in ethnic claims, as it embodies an ingrained faith in the actual existence of cultural difference that is necessary for mobilizing entitlement in complex societies. My stress on the constructedness of Latino ethnicity, and on the paradoxes and unintended consequences that surrounded the process I examine should be interpreted not as undermining the power of ethnicity, however ironic its effects within current struggles for entitlement, but rather as probing the complexity and difficulties of its meaning(s).

I am frequently asked about the patients in the programs. Latino program staff advanced a definition of "Latino-ness" imbued with traditions from imagined times and spaces, and attempted to represent ethnicity as a shared symbolic stock in order to exploit it for political, institutional, and psychiatric purposes. Since they were an occupational elite, their advocacy can be interpreted as an instance of elite political action. Much as Woolard (1989:8) points out, though, whatever commanding role elites may exercise in drawing from considerable material and symbolic capital in the struggles over identity politics, "masses" do not necessarily fall in blindly behind them.

Latino patients, the "masses" in this case, did not respond obediently to the deployment of manipulated symbols. Though often equivocal about their own experiences as inmates, they nevertheless could (and did) share in the production of signs of ethnicity applied in the programs; they constituted in effect a group of expert cultural critics even as they received treatment. Their displays of ambivalence and resistance, more often than not, were directed at the totalizing conditions of patienthood that surrounded

them. Their actions were aimed at manipulating their institutional situation rather than at rejecting the exercise in ethnicity construction in which they had been peremptorily involved—and whose political dimensions they recognized and exploited for their own purposes. Patients and staff were thus conspiratorially bound in enacting Latino-ness for different purposes, as differentially located social actors. In any event, in utilitarian terms the patients in the programs did seem to improve; minimally, they seemed more at ease in their ethnicized ambience.

The presence of patients in this book is somewhat blurred, however, owing to my deliberate focus on the process of identity construction and on the Latino mental health practitioners who were most accountable for generating and *imposing* the representations of ethnicity produced in the programs. A more prosaic, but methodologically relevant, reason for the patients' absence is that it was program staff who were the initial focus of my contracted research inquiry; I was thus constrained by the limits of the original evaluation project.

With the benefit of hindsight, though, it is now evident to me that what happened among the Latino patients in the programs may best be pondered through Estroff's (1981) notion of "making it crazy." According to this notion, when interacting with institutional and medical staff, mental patients engage in capitalizing strategies by exhibiting and *performing* a threshold degree of pathology, whatever their actual condition, in order to avail themselves of the resources that these staff control. That is, however they may actually feel, and whatever their insights about the drawbacks of psychotropic treatment, patients know enough to present themselves as "crazies" when interacting with mental health practitioners. Mental patients are not in the position to engage in normative relations of exchange to obtain resources from other institutions or domains within their immediate experiential context. The deinstitutionalized mental patients that Estroff worked with thus engaged in subsistence strategies by offering up their own mental disabilities to validate their participation in public mental health programs, and in exchange for care, support, and medication; as mental patients, they had no other viable capital to exchange.

Likewise, patients in the Latino programs were inescapably pressed to "make it crazy" in order to mobilize institutional resources, but also to "make it ethnic" to avail themselves of the specialized services that the Latino programs offered. Latino patients both embodied and capitalized on the construction of their own institutional personae as "crazy" and as "Latinos/ethnics." They thus cooperated with Latino staff in constituting a virtual ethnic community, but one that was permeated by psychiatric purposes and hierarchical relations of authority. Both Estroff and I worked within public institutions; our work engaged indigent and working-class patients rather

than those who could afford the privilege of individual therapy and the self-indulgent reflexivity of analysis. The situation in expensive private institutions may differ.

To reiterate, the immediate context for the production and reproduction of ideologies and practices of culture, ethnicity, and language that I address was the clinical settings in which typified ethnic representations were being mobilized. But these settings were themselves embedded in larger sociocultural contexts, however much the clinical and the psychiatric may be ideated as decultured, "objective" domains where people engage in impersonal applications of "scientific" techniques and knowledge. I try to account for the development of particular sociocultural modes of action that emerged in a highly localized process as the product of the intersection of these contexts.

Finally, I wish to note that I have always had a complex and ambivalent relation to this material. With the ascendancy of neoconservative opposition to affirmative action, minority language rights, desegregation measures, and other such disintegrative manifestations of the reemergence of long-standing and subjacent racism, it becomes a delicate scholarly enterprise to critically examine ethno-racial experiences and processes in the United States. In neoconservative discourses, spurious understandings about "culture" serve loaded agendas for establishing intrinsic inferiority as the defining characteristic of identified "others," and simultaneously assert that special treatment is unwarranted. By critiquing the essentializing representations of medicalized ethnicity—a critique intended, like the programs themselves, to advance much-needed political and institutional change—my arguments could be appropriated for precisely the opposite purpose.

The complexity of contemporary interethnic relations and processes is ironically marked by the fact that, even given the reliance on primordialism, one is still concerned with the ways in which dominant groups strategize their own cultural ascendancy and reproduction through the application of essentialized notions about culture and identity. My work has been received with reactions ranging from outright hilarity (among those who mistakenly see only naïve constructs of identity in the programs) to expectations that I should "solve" the issue by proposing a corrective agenda. In some venues I have been penalized for daring to critique such sacrosanct practices as psychology and psychiatry, and have received damning reactions from those who, because of my own identity and positioning, think me an ingrate and a quisling to the cause of ethnic activism for seemingly condemning these programs. This criticism seems to me particularly ironic when it comes from non-Latinos, since it reiterates yet another strain of racialization, that of benign paternalism. My work has also been challenged by anthropologists who hold very traditional notions about the discipline and its practices,

and condemn me for engaging in the examination of institutional situations in the United States rather than pursuing the craft in exotic places.

Faced with these conundrums, I have long anguished over the implications of further disseminating this work. What eventually persuaded me to publish were institutional experiences in which I found myself encountering similar strategies of essentializing—this time in academia, particularly (but not solely) in the struggles over legitimating ethnic studies as a viable scholarly field of knowledge and education. For too long now I have been witnessing a phenomenon that replays my own ethnographic ruminations as aspects of my analysis come to life on campus. In this instance, students enact the subject position that Latino patients occupy in my study, becoming implicated as typified presences in the struggle over institutional visibility, resources, and clout that is the animating principle in current politics of identity across multiple sociocultural domains in the United States.

This, however, is material for other analyses and other occasions. I continue to mull over the ambiguities of these politics. Suffice it to say that it has been the enactment of identity wars on campus that has led me to bring this book to fruition.

[1]

"It sounds like Hispanics stereotyping other Hispanics!" — *poetry ?*

In May 1989 I was hired as senior research assistant by a university-based mental health research center in New York City to work on the evaluation of three bilingual, bicultural psychiatric programs for Latino patients. The evaluation team was headed by a sociologist and included two part-time consulting anthropologists as well as three research assistants whose work I would be supervising. At the time I joined, the three-year evaluation project was barely a year old. Though the evaluation team would be applying some quantitative methods, the evaluation was mostly ethnographic.

Although I had no experience in medical, psychological, or "applied" anthropology—the disciplinary slots into which this project at first glance seemed best to fit—I was intrigued by the possibility of doing research in the mental health field. I also needed a job to support myself, a graduate student in New York City. As an incipient anthropologist and bilingual island-born Puerto Rican with a long-ago minor in psychology and experience with closed institutions from previous legal and prison reform work, I qualified for the position. During the job interview I was informed that I would be doing fieldwork as well as supervising the research assistants in their own. Our joint task was to document the institutionalization of these specialized programs. Their implementation, it was expected, would eventually produce "culturally sensitive" modalities of psychiatric treatment that could be replicated in other ethnically marked programs. The "ethnicization" of mental health care would thus become accepted public policy on the basis of its medical and institutional legitimation as documented by our evaluation of these three demonstration programs.

[13]

Catching Up with the Programs

Once hired, I familiarized myself with the histories of the evaluation and of the programs by examining existing fieldnotes, proposals, memoranda, correspondence, and reports. This archival material was of two kinds: official exchanges and documents generated by local Latino mental health professionals, state and city bureaucrats, staff in the programs and in the facilities where they were sited, and former and current members of the evaluation team; and fieldnotes and supporting documents such as forms, records, and charts already generated in fieldwork.[1] The programs had been established in inpatient mental health facilities at two New York State psychiatric centers and a New York City general hospital. In addition to differences of institutional location, there were also qualitative differences, since each program cared for certain kinds of patients and had developed particular structural components, and distinctive institutional profiles.

One of the state programs—here, "Plymouth Psychiatric Center"—cared for chronic patients in need of long-term psychiatric treatment; it included a day program which was formally part of the Latino program, even though it also attended to patients from other wards in the facility. The program in the city hospital—which I call here "Jefferson Hospital"—cared for short-term, acutely ill mental patients and consisted of an inpatient ward and an outpatient clinic. The other state program—"Northern Psychiatric Center"—served patients who required intermediate care and consisted solely of an inpatient ward.

At the time, the idea of "culturally sensitive" psychiatric care was not new to health institutions in the city, the region, or the nation. Andrade (1978), Cuellar and Martínez (1984), and Dolgin, Salazar, and Cruz (1987) document some of the psychiatric programs for Latino patients that had been established during the 1970s and 1980s in cities with considerable Latino populations: San Francisco, Denver, San Antonio, and Washington, D.C. There had been short-lived programs in New York City that incorporated "folk" elements into psychiatric care; Ruiz and Langrod (1984), for example, approvingly assess a program developed in a South Bronx outpatient community health center in which *espiritistas*—characterized as "folk healers"—were recruited as assistants. So far as I know, this particular program was no longer functioning when the Latino programs discussed here were being established, but there were similar ones in the city, such as an outpatient clinic on the Lower East Side which incorporated Latino cultural issues in family counseling and treatment (Reyes and Inclán 1991). Harwood's (1977) classic ethnography gives extensive treatment of the application of "folk" systems of belief (*santería* and *espiritismo*) in community programs.

But the programs we were evaluating constituted the first local attempts to implement culturally specific care especially for *inpatient* populations. More important, they were explicitly entrusted with the systematic development of modes of "culturally sensitive" psychiatric assessment and treatment that could potentially alter dominant psychiatric practices. As far as I could ascertain, the older programs, though entrusted with providing "culturally sensitive" care, were not specifically committed to the lofty goal of fostering change in mainstream mental health care practices. In this sense, the three pilot programs were viewed and defined—especially by those involved in their establishment—as progressive vehicles for change—although others considered them subversive of an established order.

The Political Contestation of Ethnicity

It was quite evident to me at the outset that the need for these programs was neither self-evident nor taken for granted. Their establishment required a process of negotiation, mostly driven by efforts mobilized by a local organization of Latino mental health professionals in order to persuade city and state mental health agencies of their benefits. The notion of creating special psychiatric facilities for Latinos was controversial, as was the concept of cultural sensitivity. Ironically, both concept and programs were perceived as discriminatory, representing preferential treatment for a particular ethnic group. This is, of course, anathema in policy making since preferential treatment violates public mandates of equality, derived from the U.S. Constitution itself, in the delivery of health care—especially in the case of facilities funded and operated by the state. The programs were also cynically viewed as the product of self-interested strategies on the part of Latino mental health professionals to enhance their own job prospects and political goals. Last, though certainly not least, cultural sensitivity seemed to breach psychiatric principles of universality and rationality. Objections to the programs were not organized strictly along ethno-racial lines: many Latino mental health professionals themselves feared that the establishment of the programs would result in the ghettoization of Latino patients, resulting in inferior care, and that their own participation in the effort would marginalize them as practitioners who cared only for "their own people."

Our evaluation represented an effort to legitimize the programs, and thereby cultural sensitivity, in organizational, political, and medical terms. But program advocates themselves had initiated the legitimation of cultural sensitivity by placing language at the core of their arguments: that is language difference was the decisive criterion that led to the success of the negotiations and ultimately to the establishment of the programs. These

[15]

advocates represented Latinos as predominantly Spanish speakers, and they depicted this (presumed) radical language difference as an indisputable fact that impeded the adequate delivery of mental health care for Latino patients. The proponents of the programs (justifiably) argued that monolingual patients simply could not understand therapeutic and other interactions conducted in a language foreign to them. Bilingualism, they acknowledged, did not rule out mutual incomprehension. Nevertheless, although the effect of bilingual competence on the expression of psychological symptoms was a debated issue, advocates for the programs invoked a body of research arguing for something that I began to think of as linguistic "regression": the characterization of Latino bilinguals as recurring to their native language, *assumed to be Spanish*, in moments of psychological stress. Linguistic competence in Spanish was thus incorporated as an essential *therapeutic* component of mental health practice for treating both monolingual and bilingual Latinos.

Cultural difference, by contrast was strategically minimized during the negotiations. The intersection of culture and psychiatry was a more complex matter to articulate. Underplaying culture allowed the negotiating parties to sidestep the reality of Latino diversity—the differences in origin, history, dialects, and migration experience that characterize the various Latino communities in the city and in the nation. Thorny issues of race and class could thus be glossed over as well. In addition stressing cultural difference would have undermined the efforts to establish the programs because it could have fostered similar claims from other groups. After all, the highly diverse population of New York City includes many English-speaking constituencies that consider themselves culturally dissimilar to the imagined dominant white Anglo culture. Effacing cultural issues institutionally simplified the establishment of the Latino programs: they could be portrayed as identical to ordinary programs except that the people involved in them, staff and patients, would be able to speak Spanish to one another in the course of everyday life and for therapeutic purposes. A language barrier as "objective" condition was a more palatable argument for program advocates to deploy and administrators to digest; establishing the programs would entail less ideological, bureaucratic, and budgetary upheaval if "cultural" matters were given short shrift.

In spite of these considerations, however, cultural elements were incorporated into the programs' final design—an ironic indication of the complexities entailed in articulating notions about culture. This is apparent in the programs' use of "bicultural" in their official designation and was actualized in their organizational and developmental goals: the use of Spanish for everyday and therapeutic interactions; the creation of an ethnicized environment for the patients through Latino music, art, recreation, food, and

celebrations; and the development of culturally sensitive modalities of psychiatric care. These three elements simultaneously constituted the programs' goals and their developmental schema as set forth in the proposal that their advocates submitted.

The evaluation design, in turn, addressed three parallel processual aspects in the programs' institutionalization. The evaluation team was mandated to document and assess the organization and implementation of the programs, patient and program outcomes, and the development of a conceptual model for delivering culturally sensitive mental health care to Latinos. These aspects were chronologically organized and obviously informed by the programs' goals. Thus, our first-year objective was to evaluate the implementation and organization of the programs by examining their formal and structural development and determining how successfully they had "Latino-ized" themselves by purging non-Latinos from their staff and patient populations, initiating "culturally sensitive" treatment programs, and creating a suitably ethnic ambiance. Our second-year objective was to assess the effect of this ethnicized milieu on program development and on the patients themselves as indicated by patient discharge rates and medication needs (increased discharge rates and declining need for medication are conventional indices of success in psychiatric institutions). Our third-year objective was to assess whether program staff had successfully developed culturally sensitive modalities of psychiatric care. The evaluation design was thus organized to move from examining the programs' formal and structural implementation to assessing their functional effectiveness, and culminated in appraising the more abstract goal of developing culturally sensitive psychiatric care.

In practice, of course, the evaluation fieldwork simultaneously covered all three "stages," much as did their implementation in the programs: actual life is messier than contemplated in our orderly schemes. The distinctions were barely maintained, discursively and textually, in evaluation reports. With hindsight, though, I would argue that the sequential articulation and organization of both programmatic goals and evaluation design are analytically relevant. Both constituted a conceptual scheme for "thinking" about the programs and the evaluation itself, a mental map that represented the orientation or habitus[2] characteristic among mental health professionals. Programs and evaluation were equally designed (and expected) to unfold—sequentially and linearly—and "progress" toward the lofty outcome of reconciling ethnicity ("culture") and the medical, as embodied in the articulation of rationalized, culturally sensitive modalities of care.

The programs' developmental schema and the evaluation design were thus structurally and conceptually parallel. Organized as analogous processes, they were the product of a scientistic ideological framework authorizing

how each of these events should be publicly perceived. Yet central to them was a notion of cultural sensitivity, something not typically considered in the sciences.

Valuing and Revaluing "Cultural Sensitivity"

In the assortment of proposals and research plans that sustained the establishment of the programs, the Latino professionals who were advocating for them often defined "cultural sensitivity" quite simply as the empathetic care of Latinos by Latinos. This was presented as self-evident and would become an article of faith in the implementation of the programs.

This discursive turn constituted cultural sensitivity as a statement of cultural exclusiveness, and thus invoked political relations. But those who mobilized it were also capitalizing upon ongoing debates in the psychiatric professions over widely held constructs of mental illnesses and conditions as universal phenomena properly addressed through "rational," "objective" categories of assessment and treatment (Kleinman 1988; Mezzich et al. 1996).[3] Latino practitioners were basically positing that psychiatry could be "ethnicized" by using "native" professionals to assess and treat patients in a language—Spanish—they presumably share in daily life; this would make therapeutic interactions between the two parties comprehensible and render beneficial clinical outcomes. Likewise, surrounding ethnic patients with recognizable cultural signs could ease both their psychiatric conditions and their institutional experience, contribute to their well-being, and eventually effect their "cure" or, minimally, assuage their illnesses. The application of culture and language in such ways, and for these purposes, would culminate in their insertion and systematization, articulated as culturally sensitive modalities of treatment, into mainstream psychiatric principles and practices. This, in sum, was the mental health argument on behalf of the programs and for their animating principle of cultural sensitivity.

But actions in life are never disengaged from the sociocultural relationships that produce them. Both the evaluation design and the programs' goals expressed an assumption that "ethnicity" as articulated through the notion of cultural sensitivity, could be objectified and incorporated into normative, models of psychiatric care. Entrusted with this process would be "native" Latino staff who could deploy their own cultural and linguistic knowledge for such purposes. But I found it quite telling with regard to the paradoxes involved that, among other implementation activities, the programs were required to train Latino staff in their own "culture" as a specialized domain of knowledge. Program advocates were thus configuring cul-

tural knowledge as a form of cognition that had to be isolated and labeled, then infused into mainstream psychiatric concepts and practices in order to be validated.

As I became increasingly immersed in the evaluation, I began to think about cultural sensitivity as an exercise in introspection by which cultural traits, attitudes, and behaviors, actions could be "uncovered" (discovered?).[4] But a chance remark by one of the Latino professionals who worked in the programs stuck in my mind and thrust me into a reconsideration of the complexities implicated in constructing ethnicity and culture within a clinical setting.

Political Agendas and Contrastive Strategies

In the summer of 1990 I was supervising our research assistants in the administration of a patient satisfaction questionnaire, one of the quantitative measures the government agencies that supervised the programs had insisted on. They viewed quantification as a corrective for the methodological "softness" that they imputed to the ethnographic methods we were applying.[5] After administering the questionnaire at Plymouth Psychiatric Center, we met with its Latino director to discuss his comments on the draft of an interim evaluation report. We rendered reports biannually, in the form of an interim and a final report each year; drafts were circulated for feedback among administrators of the facilities where the programs were situated program directors, and officials at the state and city agencies that supervised the facilities, as well as other selected individuals.[6]

Program staff on the front lines, so to speak, would often confidentially complain to us that they never saw our reports, were unclear on what the evaluation covered, and were unfamiliar with its findings. This experience is common in program evaluation work—which is, after all, an inherently political exercise (Cook and Shadish 1986)—because evaluators' relationship to the institutional hierarchy is differentially construed. Especially for those on the bottom rungs who are actually implementing a program's everyday tasks, evaluation can imply a kind of judgmental surveillance that they believe may affect their livelihood. This belief is not totally unfounded, since evaluations inform administrative policy and practical decisions which may be interpreted as unfair by different segments of the institution's work force. These perceptions are played out in the relations between evaluators and those evaluated, creating tension but also generating strategies to manage evaluation outcomes. Complaints such as those that were conveyed to us are strategic manifestations of resistance to the power with which evalu-

[19]

ators are invested, perceived as they often are as agents for management and as producers of a kind of knowledge to which lower level staff, believe they have no access, or feel they cannot control.

We would discuss with program administrators their responses to report drafts, responses *ideally* culled from all program staff. This process of mutual feedback, in which factual and analytical indications and conclusions were debated, generally had three possible outcomes for the final version of our reports: we could incorporate the issues raised, clarify or rectify information, or let what we had written stand as it was. This procedure repeatedly provoked instances of heated dissent and hostility, underscoring the ambivalence toward the evaluation and us as evaluators.

Writing the reports was not, strictly speaking, one of my assigned tasks, but since I was called upon to help draft and revise their content and form, I had a degree of authorial input, as well as an intermediary role in the process of feedback and comment. Research assistants were also consulted about alleged factual or interpretive discrepancies in the process of drafting and producing reports.

In contention at this particular meeting in 1990 was a section of the document in which we reported on the "progress" achieved by each program in developing cultural sensitivity. This was a point of ferocious competition among staff in the programs, precisely because the articulation of culturally sensitive modalities of care constituted for them the highest conceptual level of program development. My fieldnotes from the meeting read as follows:

> Thirdly, Ramón said that there was some stuff he didn't understand in [a particular report] section. . . . He started going through [it] . . . until he came upon the statement that "Neither Jefferson nor Plymouth have incorporated [cultural issues] into staff discussion. . . ." He went on to read out loud the part on Plymouth. Basically, his concern is that he had assumed that they *had* incorporated cultural issues into therapy. . . . We embarked upon a discussion about the matter. . . .
>
> I started by pointing out that a very important part of our task was to systematize their experience so as to develop a model for culturally sensitive care that could be replicated by other programs. I tried very hard to convey to him that we weren't attacking the quality of care at Plymouth or the extent to which there is a sense of ethnic identity among the staff which they share with the patients and the ways they use this cultural knowledge in dealing with them. Neither were we trying to set up competition among the programs. I hit upon what I hoped was an example to illustrate what the third stage entails: What if they hired a young acculturated T[herapy] A[ide] with no experience in dealing with their still mostly monolingual, native-raised, elderly population? How could they convey to this person what was expected in the ward in

treating this kind of patient? How could they train this person [to be culturally sensitive] (and Ramón, nodding, actually completed my thought even before I could finish it)?

Ramón asked me point blank what it was that they had done at Northern and I told him that the information we had was that they had gone through this whole process of consciously trying to identify cultural elements that were involved in the patients' behavior and how they manifested themselves within the institutional context, etc. Ramón mused that his experience is that they do use this kind of knowledge in dealing with their patients but that he could see how difficult it could be to articulate and systematize. I replied that it wasn't easy precisely because there is a lot of culture that appears to us to be unconscious. At one point [in our discussion] Ramón laughingly remarked that it sounded *"like Hispanics stereotyping other Hispanics."*

It did, and it was. Typification can be—and is—one of those "contrastive strategies" (Sollors 1986:27–28) formulated and deployed to legitimate the erection of ethnic boundaries of belonging. But the remark underscored the complexities involved in mobilizing unexamined representations of Latino culture within the context of the programs.

The representations of Latino ethnicity that were being produced, as I have already noted, constituted the means for Latino mental health professionals to gain control over "technologies of power" and medical services (Greenwood et al. 1988:1). Latino professionals were conscious that they were not in the position, as migrant (or immigrant) others in a dominant host culture, to control thoroughly these institutionalized systems of health care delivery.

Yet the arguments used to persuade government officials to stamp their imprimatur on the programs were organized around depictions of Latino culture that emphasized its otherness in the United States. Latinos were being homogenized as natives of traditional agrarian cultures who suffer as a result of multiple cultural and linguistic barriers that block their access to adequate mental health care; to compound this situation, migration was viewed, in and of itself, as a stressor that exacerbated or even produced mental illness. Latino professionals were characterizing *the* Latino interactional style as warm and caring, in opposition to the perceived coldness and impersonality of both the institutional environment and the host culture. While they acknowledged Latino bilingualism, they also emphasized Spanish monolingualism as a pervasive mark of identity, and thus of otherness; bilinguals were portrayed as linguistically disadvantaged in therapeutic settings whatever their actual communicative competence. These representations were being advanced by Latinos who could claim expert knowledge in the matter on the strength of their dual identity as Latinos and as mental health professionals. Their portrayals were neither totally explicit nor con-

sistent, but were woven through a discourse of difference that was often contradicted by the conditions that prevailed in the programs.

These were the political uses of ethnicity. But within the medical settings in which the programs were sited, these cultural representations took on the quality of a typified knowledge that had to be systematized along the lines of a psychiatric discourse and its attendant practices. Ethnic consciousness—how people understand and use ethnicity—had to be made explicit, become objectified, and be articulated with psychiatric models.[7] Configured as a form of cognition that could be decontextualized and isolated, ethnicity would then be amenable to transfer beyond the site of its production within the relations obtaining in the programs (cf. Lave 1988:9, 40ff.). The evolutionistic design common to both the programs' developmental schema and the evaluation plan, describing a gradual trajectory of "progress" culminating in the insertion of ethnic elements into standard modalities of psychiatric treatment, reinforced the positivistic quality of these figurations about ethnicity.

My associates who devised the evaluation plan shared a strong clinical orientation with the programs' advocates. In the research center's work, "cultural sensitivity" was a major construct articulated in terms of psychological and psychiatric notions, but it was not explicitly defined except as entailing accessibility to treatment, the modification of treatment modalities, or the transformation of patients' behavior or attitudes. Cultural difference—defined as anything not pertaining to a dominant "Anglo" culture, itself a vague and contestable proposition—was seen as a condition that impeded access to mental health care and automatically rendered psychiatric treatment inefficacious. Migration was assumed to produce cultural dissonance and personal stress which became major etiological factors in the incidence of mental conditions among the culturally "different." Although some at the research center would protest my interpretation, their approach to ethnicity and mental health care implicitly reproduced the formulations and constructs that underlay the programs.

What ostensibly made our evaluation project different from other research at the center was the use of ethnography and the attempt to draw from anthropological frames of understanding in assessing the programs. It was a difficult fit, though, because of the functionalist assumptions in both the evaluation plan and the programs' developmental schema. Whereas a more refined anthropological framework might situate "culture" in the relations obtaining among patients and staff in the programs, in these medical contexts culture was reduced to content. This reduction also eliminated any possibility of reading culture against the larger context of the experience of Latinos or their subject relations with U.S. society—except, perhaps, in terms of migration myths that are largely foreign to them.

Yet I began to recognize how the representations about culture, ethnicity, and language produced by these Latino professionals could be seen as local definitions and models drawn from those that commonly circulate in U.S. society, being strategically articulated and mobilized within a medical setting. The political dimensions of the programs were and are patent, but the strategies for their establishment and validation had to be accommodated to an assimilating medical ideology and practice as well as to common definitions about ethnicity, however essentializing they might be.

Significantly, the cultural demographics in the programs were not that simple. There were large proportions of Puerto Ricans and "Nuyoricans"—U.S.-born or raised Puerto Ricans—among patients and staff, whose presence sometimes gave the programs a certain deceptive homogeneity that was actually fragmented by an increasing influx of natives from other countries. These "newer" Latino patients (and mental health practitioners) reflected the trend of Latino migration into New York City, particularly since the 1970s, which encompassed a varied array of personal histories, national cultures and identities, migration experiences, and dialectal forms of Spanish. Such intra-Latino diversity further negated the conflation of different national and cultural groups under the monolithic representations of "Hispanicity" or "Latino-ness" that program staff were constructing. The programs were increasingly populated with young, urban- and U.S.-born, bilingual and even English-monolingual Latino patients—youths whose histories, social experiences, and behaviors were obviously not those of the idealized (and ideated) monolingual native of a "traditional" Latino society which so monologized the local representations.

Program staff exhibited a similar diversity. Moreover, a shortage of Latino mental health professionals and paraprofessionals defeated the programmatic goal of totally Latino staffing; the shortage was compounded by the disincentives for working in public health facilities serving the indigent. The recruitment of non-Latinos to work in the programs introduced an additional array of identities and experiences to be negotiated. Likewise, the hierarchical relations that obtain in mental health institutions between professional and paraprofessional staff at one level, and between staff and patients at another, inserted elements of class difference that further fragmented the homogeneity expected to prevail within the programs.

The gaps between model and experience, along with the degree of typification marshaled to validate the Latino programs, led me to reconsider my perceptions about the process I was witnessing. I began to focus on how Latino program staff engaged in an exercise of cultural and ethnic definition in the production of "selves" (Goffman 1959) to be presented to agencies, patients, and researchers for the legitimation of political, social, and economic ends. My analyses were increasingly informed by the ways in which

[23]

issues of cultural and linguistic difference were addressed in specific contexts, but also how they reiterated the treatment of cultural difference in the United States in general, where it has become a core cultural construct. The analysis of difference has generated a vast scholarly literature from which I chose in order to guide my examination.

Why "Ethnicity"?

The simple answer to the question "Why 'ethnicity'?" is that I use the term "ethnicity" rather than "race" because this is what the people I worked with preferred. Beyond the importance of respecting the "natives," though, it is analytically useful to subsume the idea of race into that of ethnicity, but without overlooking the racializing manner in which particular identities are treated in discursive formations and strategies, in order to address the insertion of Latino culture into medical and institutional domains that are typically imagined as decultured fields of action.

It has become a commonplace to note that both ethnicity and race are sociocultural constructs. As such, they challenge universalistic notions of personhood inscribed in the dominant ideological schema of individualism that emerged, particularly in the United States, under conditions of modernity. In accounting for the apparent waxing of ethnicity in recent decades,[8] Sollors (1986:20–21; 1996:xviff.) points out that most social science theorizing about the concept to that time was anchored by "expectations"—ideological, cultural, and political—that such "tribalistic" traits (predicating identity and allegiance based on "ethnicity" and "race") would disappear with the coalescing of modern, universalistic, and technocratic societies around the world. This was especially anticipated after the demise of totalitarian nationalisms that espoused notions of ethno-racial superiority which contributed to the disasters of the Second World War. Postwar theorists argued that class would (perhaps) be the only remaining grounds for identity construction in modern societies. It is obvious by now, however, that issues of cultural difference have not been so tractable, and its descriptors and manifestations, articulated as ethno-racial identity, remain salient.

Underscoring the phenomenon's paradoxical malleability is Barth's (1969) classic definition of ethnicity as a process of identity construction that emerges in intercultural contact and persists in spite of interaction and interdependence among different cultural groups, labile participation in the affairs of these groups, and the flow of persons across ethnic boundaries. Given the persistence of ethnicity and its ambiguity, it is necessary to address the specific historicity and locality of ethnic processes to under-

stand their constitution. Here I am concerned with Latino identity and its relation to institutional discourses and practices in the United States, focusing on how this identity is manifested within medical and bureaucratic domains in the delivery of public health services. This is not a simple, coherent process but one fraught with the paradoxes generated whenever social actors engage in strategies of cultural production and reproduction, especially from conditions of structural inequality. Although the mental health practitioners I worked with could be characterized as an ethnic elite and thus structurally differentiated from the people on whose behalf they spoke and acted, they remained "ethnics" who, in spite of their occupational mobility and achievement of authority, still indexed subordinate social locations.

Thus, like Comaroff (1992, 1996), I conceive ethnicity as emanating from relations of inequality among culturally defined groups, expressed and practiced in the intercultural encounters of everyday life through the deployment of material and symbolic signs. Ethnic identity, as he argues, becomes "naturalized" when it acquires contextual saliency in the experiences of the social actors who claim it. It may then be sustained by conditions, different from those that produced it. Unlinked from its originating structural and historic conditions, ethnicity acquires a quality of timelessness, tangibility, and reality that primordializes it, rendering it an experience of cultural difference that is perceived in terms of its own self-validating autonomy (Wilmsen 1996). But ethnic identities often embody and retain sets of attributes that mark those who claim it as members of structurally subjugated groups.

This processual outcome, by which ethnicity becomes a sustained and sustainable expression of cultural difference as well as a marker for differentially valued identities, has allowed it to acquire an equivocal yet pervasive aura in the United States that fosters its typification and reduction. Ethnicity has become a requisite component of personal and collective identity that we are all expected to acknowledge, embrace, and apply at different levels of social interaction: in our everyday engagements with others; in generating representations of the self for public institutional purposes; and in the reconstitution of the nation as an interlocking identity grid by which groups of people may be defined, located, and contained.

Ethnicity now occupies a pivotal role in the redistribution of material and symbolic resources in the United States, a process understood as emanating from principles of civic entitlement and egalitarian inclusion. It has thus acquired a crucial role in structuring sociocultural experience and relations, since the nation exists in the tense interstices between claims of cultural diversity and homogenizing assimilationism, and between a collectivizing communalism and a universalizing individualism. As I see it, this applies

[25]

even through the very negation or erasure of ethnicity. It is this tension that here informs my analysis of cultural and linguistic difference in the United States.

In sum, claims to ethnicity in the United States are subject to public affirmation in a context of contradictory ideological principles and cultural practices that attempt to reconcile ethnic diversity with idealized homogeneity. The historical and sociocultural weight attributed to ethnicity fosters the production of strategies of manipulation and management, constituting forms of sociocultural action devised to alter systemic constraints (Domínguez 1986:12). Ethnicity within the United States becomes a territorially, culturally, or historically bounded construct mobilized by means of contrastive strategies (Sollors 1986:27–28). Social actors use these strategies to mark a kind of in-group membership that is constituted as sociocultural reality. A constructed reality then intersects with class, gender, and the collective and individual histories of the people who devise and advance it; ethnicity is both constitutive of relations and constituted through relations. The contrastive strategies point to sets of differentiating dispositions and practices that trigger a sense of uniqueness.

These are hardly new observations. But in the Latino programs that I worked with, I saw the iteration of a strong and persistent monism that is characteristic of the manner in which ethnicity is too often dealt with in the United States. There is a degree of practical and discursive consciousness (Giddens 1979:5) in the ways in which ethnicity indexes complex specificities of history, experience, and social location. But this consciousness is tempered by the countering pull of dominant narratives that retain the play between homogeneity and difference as a core sociocultural construct and normative practice.

Yet another layer of complexity is added in the case of Latinos given their multivalent histories both in general and as a *racialized* group in the United States. Latino diversity challenges the dominant black/white dichotomy which authorizes polarized notions about cultural difference and erases Latino specificity.[9] In response to these complexities, some Latino sectors advocate using "race" as the preferred construct, particularly when issues of power are involved, precisely because it fits well with the prevailing black/white dichotomy, exploiting and capitalizing on it.

The problems in using "race," though, are demonstrated in just such exercises. Omi and Winant (1994) are among those who advocate for the centrality of race, given the history of intercultural relations in the United States. But their analysis is an instructive example of how the unproblematized characterization of Latinos as a "race" becomes reductionistic and fails to do justice to the complexity of the Latino experience. While I agree that a hegemonic racial order exists here, I take it as a departure point rather

than as an explanatory construct and analytic end in and of itself. Characterizing the choice of "ethnicity" rather than "race" as politically conservative, as Omi and Winant do, is unproductive. As Darder and Torres (1998:9) point out, embracing the "race" paradigm was viable political strategy for Latinos in its time, and may still be for particular purposes, but "ethnicity" is not intrinsically dissonant with radical political agendas.

Particularly relevant to any analysis involving local politics of identity in New York City, a context in which both Latinos and African Americans are leading players, is that those who propose using "race" as category du jour for all culturally differentiated groups in the United States overlook the power of the white/black dichotomy. The prevalence of black-white binomialism renders "Latino/a" an ambiguous identity, given its histories of racial mixture. Reinserting Latinos into this racial dichotomy would contribute to diluting their difference vis-à-vis other contending cultural groups in the nation.[10]

I prefer to approach Latino ethnicity as the dynamic and manifold phenomenon it is rather than reduce it to a question of "choice," as often happens with identity processes in the United States. "Latino" emerged as a differentially positioned identity in the context of a history of relations characterized by colonialist and neocolonialist ideologies and strategies instantiated in actual historic circumstances: the Monroe Doctrine, western expansion, the Mexican American and Spanish American wars, the multiple military occupations of various Latin countries—hemispheric interventionist diplomacy in general. An overdetermined "Latino" category of identity indexes these historical conditions as well as the profound racialization of the diverse nationalities and local communities as they were differentially incorporated into the nation's sociocultural structures (Steinberg 1989). "Latino-ness" has been inscribed in a variety of contexts through a multiplicity of signs in myriad urban and rural spaces throughout the United States over several centuries, and is now institutionalized within a national grid of identity, paradigmatic in the U.S. census, and authorized in a multiplicity of sociocultural domains as a dubious marker of inclusion. Even before the turn toward multiculturalism, claims to ethnicity have thus acquired symbolic capital to determine institutional entitlement. "Latino-ness" enters national discourses and experiences as a concrete entity now authorized by a newly articulated "multiculturalist" order, seemingly unmoored from the historic relations and social locations that generated it.

In grappling with the ambiguities of the race/ethnicity dichotomy in the United States, I found productive Urciuoli's elaboration of both constructs. She stresses the semiotic and indexical nature of identity constructs, arguing that "race" and "ethnicity," rather than being the concrete, self-evident "facts" they are popularly imagined to be in the United States, are actually

"constructions of difference opposed to each other in complex ways," which implicate a history of a national discourse about "difference, value, and belonging" (1996:15). As constructs, race and ethnicity can then be examined in the realm of dynamic discursive practices, provided we take care to avoid their essentialization as real and timeless positions occupied by groups of people by virtue of phenotype, history, national origin, language, customs, and other such "traits." Racializing and ethnicizing discourses render problematic the simple mapping of a nature/culture dichotomy onto race and ethnicity, and underscore their conflation with class produced in the formation of the nation-state and consequent validation myths of purity and belonging (Williams 1989, 1991). Urciuoli writes:

> Racial and ethnic discourses make up the myths of purity in the nation-state. Racialized people are typified as human matter out of place: dirty, dangerous, unwilling, or unable to do their bit for the nation-state. In ethnic discourses, cultural difference is safe, ordered, a contribution to the nation-state offered by striving immigrants making their way up the ladder of class mobility. (1996:15)

Within this categorical array, a generic white English-speaking "American" emerges as an unmarked category and normative standard for all sociocultural purposes, while the alternative identities—perceived as nonnormative—constitute marked categories that become embodied in the twin constructs of race and ethnicity. But because the contrast is a politicized rather than a "natural" one, ethnicity and race are then culturally constituted as poles of an identity continuum ranging from "slightly marked [as different] and *safely* different to highly marked and *dangerous*" (1996:17; my emphasis). In this semiotic array, ethnicity is allocated to the "safe" pole, while race occupies the opposite, dubious pole of "danger." Thus signified, the two constructs become discursive markers of difference deployed to differential sociocultural effect. Vis-à-vis the unmarked "white American" category, though, *both* ethnicity and race remain markers of exclusion.

We thus walk a fine line, using cultural constructs that should not be reified to locate groups of people in differential positions within existing power structures. Though I appreciate the arguments made by scholars such as Omi and Winant (1994), particularly their articulation of the notion of a hegemonic racial formation in the United States, I also believe that the analytical productivity of "race" is compromised for several reasons. First, subsuming all identities under it is reductive. Second, race is a construct that variably informs Latino identity; Latino "racial" complexity, after all, makes the population conceptually and pragmatically interesting. Third,

and to return to my starting point, an anthropological agenda requires that one respect one's collaborators' wishes of self-designation.

What I stress here, then, is the fact of power that shapes identity constructs and their dynamic deployment as discursive elements rather than as actual, static, reified entities. I believe that this distinction is particularly salient in the United States, where the assertion of difference collides with an ideological order of equality. What happened in the Latino mental health programs may be characterized as an attempt to engage in ethnicizing discourses directed toward revaluing a racialized Latino identity. But the two discursive formations coexist and circulate together. Indeed, the interplay of racializing and ethnicizing discourses is aptly exemplified in the characterization of "culture" as a psychopathogenic factor among Latinos—a racialized assertion—but also as a palliative for inequality and for psychic and sociocultural disjuncture. A homogenized, typified Latino culture is thus rendered as the ethnicized source of redeeming cozy traditions and customs.

Methodological Considerations

Although I draw from data produced in the evaluation, this book does not duplicate the findings the evaluation team eventually generated. Some of the points we made correlate with several I address here, but the analytical modes and purposes are different. The evaluation was strongly instrumental and political, formally designed to produce recommendations that could be implemented by administrators, systematized within the programs, and replicated in other ethnically marked mental health programs; it was also entrusted with a political mandate to legitimate the programs. We were conscious of this fact and therefore of the delicacy of our task, and were particularly reminded of it when we were critical of any aspect of the programs.

More important, my analysis goes beyond the parameters of the evaluation objectives as defined in the developmentalist framework contemplated in its design (however much this may have been violated in practice). As I began to encounter the paradoxes generated in the processes of negotiation and conciliation engaged in by the participants in the programs, my research agenda became more open-ended. I spent the last year of evaluation in particular doing "double duty," so to speak, feeling torn when I engaged in evaluation work along the evolutionistic lines that had been drawn and mulling over what underpinned them. The inevitable outcome generated criticism, however diplomatic or unconscious, when some evaluation team members thought that I was diverging too far from our boundaries and be-

[29]

coming too critical in my examination of the modes of identity construction that were being generated in the Latino programs.

Ironically, one of the most persuasive criteria for my recruitment into the evaluation team was my ethnicity. Consonant with the identity constructs being deployed at the programs, being a member of the tribe would presumably imbue me with the appropriate knowledge and "cultural sensitivity" to discover, identify, and analyze how staff at the programs were (or were not) addressing "cultural" issues and needs. The very structures of understanding that were being applied to and within the programs thus ostensibly needed to be replicated in the evaluation team, and were visited on me—proof of their pervasiveness.

The research assistants—with a single exception, all Latinos—and I were pigeonholed in this way as the "native" researchers, presumed to have special insight into the "cultural" strategies we were assessing. At first I did not question the assumption, even finding something vaguely humorous in it, especially since, living in the United States as an identifiable "other," one becomes quite familiar with the essentializing that undergirds such typecasting. My own situation indexed the complex debates that prevailed in the programs and informed my analyses, articulating with local essentialist models of identity construction. At another level, it also articulated with larger questions about doing anthropology in the United States— those enervating debates over whether one's own society is an appropriate subject of anthropological inquiry and who is authorized to engage in it.

My research and professional situation, then and now, thus foregrounds questions of power that are endemic in disciplinary practices: current challenges to doing "native" anthropology generally emerge (and stick) when the anthropologist in question is also perceived and identified as a member of an ethnic group. The ambiguity surrounding my own Puerto Rican identity complicated (and still complicates) these difficult issues (cf. Lassalle and Pérez 1997). As an island-born and raised Puerto Rican anthropologist doing fieldwork in the United States, examining processes of identity construction intrinsic to the nation's self-definitional strategies, I violate essentialistic notions concerning the construction of "Latino-ness," as well as debates about the appropriateness of subjecting the United States to the anthropological "gaze," especially the "gaze" of an exotic "other." Perhaps as Latino anthropologists we need to stress that there is no such geographic entity as Latinoland—except as culturally construed loci within the United States from which emanate a particular attributed identity.

As a practical matter, both occupational training and my own life script distanced me from the Latino mental health practitioners I worked with. However much of my own cultural knowledge I self-consciously brought to

bear on the data, my immediate ethnographic context was always the clinical setting in which the programs were established and the process of their institutionalization, a domain that was familiar yet also ideologically, epistemologically, and experientially distant from me.

It was clear, too, that the mental health practitioners at the program acknowledged my identity as a Puerto Rican and fellow Latina. This allowed me to constitute for myself relations that were quite different from those that were being constituted for me as a member of an evaluation team. The bottom line is that my status as both insider and outsider simultaneously facilitated and aggravated the intrinsically oxymoronic task of participant observation (see Aguilar 1981).

Among the parameters hewn by the evaluation agenda, yet another shaped both my fieldwork and its textualization here: much of the data was generated as a team effort. In this book I have drawn from material produced by other researchers before and after my recruitment, treating earlier data as archival and historical material that gave me a context on which to build; these data complemented my own, further thickening my observations and analyses. I should also note that the data ranged further than I do here: this book is constructed out of a far larger universe of data that covered a multiplicity of quotidian aspects in program implementation and administration which I only partially summarize, if I address them at all.

Woven through other researchers' fieldnotes and reports I found overarching themes about the institutionalization of the programs reiterated in and by my own. Because of my supervisory position, I discussed data with all other members of the evaluation team: we triangulated. What emerged during these discussions was not necessarily collected or recorded in written form, but it informed my analyses. It constitutes what Ottenberg (1990:144ff.) characterizes as "headnotes": data that subsist in our minds, but are often more significant and productive than the objectified jottings we perpetuate in actual written fieldnotes.

We engaged in participant observation as well as informal and formal interviewing. Most of the interviews were informal and open-ended, or even the everyday verbal interactions that are part of effective participant observation. We also devised an interview protocol at the end of the evaluation period to guide the elicitation of uniform information from paraprofessionals in the programs about their linguistic, ethnic, and occupational experiences. One of the most vexing aspects of the research stemmed from program staff's resistance to audiotaping, particularly among the professionals. With few exceptions, none of the activities or talks with staff or patients were taped; they could only be perpetuated in fieldnotes, most as para-

phrased discourses. A good deal of valuable linguistic data was thus irre-
trievable except as paraphrase—and thus the predominance of paraphrase
in my documentation. What appears as direct quotation was noted down in
situ or is drawn from the few interactions we managed to tape.

The attitude toward taping was impressed upon me in one of my first interviews with a Puerto Rican psychiatrist. My request to tape was granted
politely but with ill-concealed displeasure. Caught between the dilemma of
gathering reliable data and accommodating her, I opted for taping, hoping
to overcome her resistance eventually. The tape recorder lay on the table
between us, but she consistently avoided acknowledging its presence. After
a series of questions that were answered routinely, sometimes hostilely and
shallowly, I leaned over and turned off the tape recorder. The psychiatrist
perked up and told me, "*¡Ahora que apagaste esa porquería, podemos
hablar de verdad!*" (Now that you've turned off that piece of junk, we can
really talk!). *Porquería* is used in Spanish to describe an object of little value
but connotes as well such polluting qualities as indecency, filth, grossness,
even obscenity, all of which she was indexing and attributing to the deceptively neutral technology of taping. (In some contexts the blandest collo-
quial English equivalent would be "crap" or "shit.") But once I turned off
the tape recorder, she really talked to me.

Staff legitimated their avoidance of taping by appealing to the confidentiality that attaches to therapeutic relationships. But a significant point for
me was that they invoked confidentiality on behalf of the patients as concerned guardians of their privacy and well-being—even though it was the
program staff who were really our targeted informants. Confidentiality was
thus articulated as a way of protecting patients as producers of utterances
that they ostensibly owned but in this instance were actually being controlled by staff. Ironically, then, this strategy further divested patients of
features of "normality" such as mobility, privacy, and agency that enable sociocultural actors to engage in effective linguistic production. What I am
suggesting is that the injunction on taping was not merely a methodological
issue, a hindrance to the production and collection of research data; it also
points out the paradoxes involved in the differential relationships that govern clinical settings. As happens in other closed institutions, the barriers of
contact and communication between inmates and the outer world were
being established, controlled, and mobilized through institutional hierarchies. Yet the resocializing purpose that ostensibly informs institutional
treatment is predicated on inmates' autonomy and their manifestation of
the will to self-correction. Once again, even in the generation of data presumably directed toward benefiting the programs, tropes of power were
manifest.

[32]

The "Medical"

Finally, I wish to address the place of this work vis-à-vis medical anthropology. I address the medical as a cultural realm, particularly in the chapters that document the actual conditions, ideologies, and practices that obtained in the programs. I stress how their actual operations constituted them as moral, and not natural, systems (Evans-Pritchard 1962). Since the programs were designed for Latino patients, my focus is necessarily on how these mental health practitioners, engaged in assessing behavior and construing it in particular ways, contributed to the reconstitution of Latinos, not only as a group but also as stereotypical sociocultural personae. Psychiatrists and psychologists engage in determining a person's ability to participate in parity with others in a society; in the present case, this complex exercise was compounded by the boundaries of participation that have been differentially drawn for Latinos and their communities. Generally, psychiatry and medicine determine what is adequate or normal or appropriate or true, and thus engage in moral assessments about people and relations. I argue that staff in the Latino programs deployed occupational knowledge and modes of behavior in order to validate sociopolitical action, but also contributed to the production of notions about Latinos and Latino culture that authorized unfavorable—and pathologizing—comparisons between them and an imagined "mainstream" Anglo-American culture.

The relationship between anthropology and psychiatric beliefs and practices has always been complex and ambivalent. For example, Sapir (1949:514) recognized the tensions between them, revolving around the skepticism anthropologists display—or *should* display—toward acknowledging as legitimate notions such as "normal behavior" which are among the most valued psychiatric constructs.

The concept of normality in the Latino programs became ambiguous because their institutionalization mandated the articulation of "culture" with psychiatry, two culturally differentiated ideations of what the normal should be. I follow contemporary trends of critical analysis in examining the process. But I also underscore that my focus is ethnicity, and not so much the medical per se. I thus engage in an examination of how structural and institutional principles and practices within a medical-clinical domain impinge on everyday "micro" conditions. My analyses are strongly informed by a Foucaultian perspective (1965, 1972, 1977, 1978, 1980) as well as contemporary critiques of the medical realm, particularly Gaines (1985, 1992), Good (1994), Hahn (1995), Hahn and Gaines (1985), Hahn and Kleinman (1983), Kleinman (1985, 1988, 1995), Lindenbaum and Lock (1993), Marsella and White (1982), Petersen and Bunton (1997), and Zola (1986).

There is an extensive body of literature addressing the situation of Latinos within the mental health field,[11] a subset that points to a long-standing multidisciplinary concern with complexities in the relationship between mental illness and its treatment, on the one hand, and ethno-racial identity and class, on the other. In this literature, subordinate class positions and ethno-racial identity are consistently associated with high rates of mental illness (e.g., Dohrenwend and Dohrenwend 1969; Hollingshead and Redlich 1958; Myers and Bean 1968; Special Populations 1978), an orientation, to my way of thinking, that is probably more revealing of psychiatric categories, differential positioning, racialization, and institutional practices than of the actual situation, since these descriptors are contingent on sociocultural principles of "normality." The association between class and ethno-racial identity reflects the conflation of cultural difference and class that, as Urciuoli (1996) and Williams (1986) argue, contributes to the politics of identity in the United States.

In addressing cultural difference, medical anthropology has tended to document clusters of behavior deemed to be culturally defined and specific as "folk" categories of psychiatric conditions. Harwood (1981) represents this trend when he summarizes native concepts of illness and disease as explanatory constructs that biomedical practitioners must consider in order to treat cultural "others" effectively. The repertoire of mental conditions among Latinos usually addressed include *susto* and *ataque de nervios*, both of which have been sanctioned as culture-bound syndromes, are described in the literature as legitimate manifestations of psychic distress within the context of standard cultural principles and practices, and have been recognized in the American Psychiatric Association's diagnostic manual (APA 1987, 1994). The focus on these "folk" syndromes is consonant with one of the animating principles of medical anthropology: the examination of culturally specific systems of meaning in the definition and interpretation of conditions that are perceived by members of different cultural groups as forms of illness and disease. These "folk" syndromes are thus neatly distinguished from those objectified in biomedicine—that is, Western medical categories and practices.

Nevertheless, even in the 1990s practitioners of medical anthropology were still expressing their concern that, in spite of the wealth of research into these Latino "folk" conditions, they were poorly understood and addressed by mental health institutions. More important, Latino needs, it was argued, were not being properly addressed by medical and psychiatric institutions and personnel. For example, Guarnaccia, Good, and Kleinman (1990) critically review the epidemiological studies on Puerto Rican mental health and urge that cross-cultural psychiatric studies incorporate further "indigenous categories of experience" as explored through

carefully designed research, rather than rely solely on instruments that "treat culture as a confounding variable to be controlled and eliminated" (1990:1455).

The recognition of culture-bound syndromes in *DSM-IV* (APA 1994)—though not of a fully validated "cultural axis"—potentially represents another set of issues. Guarnaccia and Rogler (1999) argue for the need to develop a "new" research agenda precisely because the perception of increased cultural diversity makes it ever more pressing that such syndromes be examined on their own terms ("within their own cultural context") rather than subsumed into existing psychiatric categories. The authors articulate their proposed research agenda as encompassing the nature of the phenomenon, the sociocultural location of its sufferers, the relationship of the syndromes to psychiatric disorders, and their social and psychiatric history within the life course of the individual. In my view, such an agenda relocates the inquiry as an empirical issue best addressed through ethnography rather than through clinical measures of assessment, which are, unfortunately, the research instruments usually brought to bear on the matter.

These critiques are apt. Generally, though, they do not address the actual conditions in which cultural knowledge is applied and how it is articulated within what is, after all, yet another cultural domain. It was abundantly evident to us during the evaluation that *susto* and *ataque de nervios*, however validated through scholarly research, were, in practice, usually "translated" into standard psychiatric categories. Thus, on at least one occasion in one of the Latino programs, an *ataque de nervios*, even when recognized as such, was discursively characterized as "hysteria" and treated through the application of a Freudian interpretive framework—that is, as a psychosexual expression of female distress.

My own work, I believe, lies closer to that which addresses the institutional and practical contexts in which health is ministered to for differentially constituted sociocultural actors (e.g., Hahn and Gaines 1985; Marsella and White 1982). That is, the clinical and the medical are intrinsically cultural domains rather than just a contextual field on which "the cultural"—be it in the form of culture-bound syndromes or as a culturally sensitive practice—can simply be placed as a separate entity without any consideration of the interactions and mutually constituting effects of all the relevant domains. Rather than engage in an examination of "folk" categories of disease or their place in psychiatric classificatory grids, I foreground the political dimensions of institutional practices and the construction of ethnicity among ethnic elites who wield cultural and professional authority within a contemporary sociocultural domain permeated with power.

[2]

Negotiating Ethnicity

Ethnic claims are often negotiated through the competition that characterizes political life in pluralistic societies. In this chapter I examine the process by which Latino mental health professionals and paraprofessionals began to construct scenarios to legitimate their claim to the Latino programs. These scenarios embody representations about Latino ethnicity that are partially predicated on the definition of Latinos as a population in need, and are then translated into the therapeutic realm in terms of group identity (Flores and Yúdice 1990:60). In addition to the political strategy of constituting Latino patients as a population in need, the representations generated during negotiations were equally informed by "commonsense" notions about Latino culture imbued with essentializing assumptions. Spanning a number of years, the negotiations over the programs acquired, for all of us who became involved in them, the resonance of a shared historic narrative and founding charter.

I use the term "charter" deliberately (Malinowski 1944), to stress how the negotiations were "sacralized." They retained an aura of authority even though many, perhaps most of us who later participated in the actual implementation of the programs, did not participate in the negotiations. For those who did, they became a source of local prestige and knowledge, constituting the participants as symbolic "tribal" elders and conferring on them an authority that was appealed to whenever problematic situations emerged in the administration of the programs. In this sense, participating in the negotiations contributed to the reproduction of internal professional hierarchies as well as to the allocation and reallocation of prestige and power among the individuals in their local occupational communities.

A series of vexing issues also emerged during the negotiations which foreshadowed those that would shape the programs' character. The negotiations thus must be examined both for a full understanding of the programs' significance, and because they illustrate how particular modes of ethnic strategizing became linked to prevailing self-representations. The process thus anticipated recurrent complexities in the polyvalent process of identity construction.

Since I did not participate in them, my account of the negotiations is mostly culled from materials elicited by other fieldworkers. Once I joined the evaluation team, I met and worked with many of the primary participants; this allowed me to further "thicken" my interpretation of the process from several vantage points. Others at the program who also had no personal knowledge of the event would often draw on it as a historicizing or framing device that enhanced the meaning, documented the importance or established the complexity of consequent developments. This underscores the signifying effects that the negotiation narrative had on participants' interpretation of their experiences of the programs.

The negotiations represented an occasion for the convergence of different, often opposed ideologies. Negotiators thought of themselves as representing divergent interests and concerns, but also as expert proponents of "solutions" for managing the practical and ideological problems entailed by the proposal for culturally sensitive care. Each of the adversarial groups in question—Latino advocates and mostly non-Latino administrators—felt that it represented a constituency that could be adversely affected by the establishment of the programs. Latino advocates constituted themselves as cultural brokers for their communities and as experts in the mental health field; administrators drew upon highly rationalized bureaucratic principles of policy making and public service delivery. Crucially at stake in this process was the production of a persuasive definition of "Latino-ness" that would legitimate the ethnicization of mental health care under the tutelage of Latino practitioners. The negotiations thus involved articulating cultural difference in ways that could override the twin rationales for uniformity: the universalizing force of psychiatric treatment, and the ideological tenets that inform its delivery in public institutions operating under a legal dictum of equality.

Locating Institutional Politics

The negotiations did not occur in a vacuum. They responded to contemporary national concerns about the management of contending ethnic interests, emerging at a particular historic juncture in which dominant cul-

tural narratives about identity, immigration, diversity, and citizenship had acquired saliency in the public discourse, and presumptions about the automatic parity of ethno-racial groups in assimilation were being overtly contested. Communities around the nation were clinging tenaciously to their own sense of cultural uniqueness, yet at the same time asserting their rights to equal public participation. The ensuing debates revolved around the extent to which representations, place, and entitlements, organized around a discourse of cultural difference, should be authorized in a society in which the yardstick of identity was (and is) still inflected through standards of whiteness and Anglicity that persist however imagined they may be.

Much in these debates has been necessarily articulated in terms of legality and the policy-making power of the state. Cultural difference brings into play questions about the integration or segregation of particular groups in the society, their access to institutional processes and services, and the potential ideological rupture that asserting entitlement on the basis of difference represents for principles of egalitarianism and individualism. Egalitarianism prescribes equality of opportunity and treatment, while individualism favors a subject-centered stance in capitalizing on institutional resources. Because of a tradition of public care in matters of mental health, the state is necessarily enmeshed in the consideration of these issues in a policy-making, jural role that informs and circumscribes (but also enables) social action. Arguing for the importance of an institutional foundation for psychiatric discourse, Fábrega (1996:6–7) foregrounds the role of state action in psychiatric practices. Like other sectors of the society, then, the state produces what Myers (1988:613) has called "interpretive scenarios," through which instances of cultural difference that it perceives as problematic are substantiated.

With regard to Latino mental health, there was one state document that generated such a scenario; its portrayal of Latinos and their health needs informed the terms in which the programs were conceptualized. The document was a report to a presidential committee created in 1977 to study the delivery of public services to African Americans, Native Americans, and Latinos. The Latino professionals involved in the negotiations indexed this textual scenario to validate the establishment of the New York programs. Further entextualized and recontextualized (Silverstein and Urban 1996) in written documents, oral arguments, and everyday discourses, this report supported their claims as it defined and represented Latinos as a population in particular need of specialized mental health services. Even after the programs were established, the report remained a text that was constantly appealed to, woven and rewoven into the discourses generated by program advocates and staff. It was part of an ideological genealogy within which

specific arguments being deployed to legitimize the concept of culturally sensitive care could be located.

Since this report took on great ideological weight, it is the first element that I examine so as to provide the context for the history of the negotiations. Authored by the Special Populations Sub-Task Panel on the Mental Health of Hispanic Americans, the report was delivered to a twenty-member President's Commission on Mental Health, which included six "minority" persons: three African Americans, two Latinos, and one Native American. Seventeen of the twenty-one members of the Sub-Task Panel were Latino mental health professionals.

A Matter of Public Concern

Lessinger (1991) points out that the concern over minorities and institutionalized mental health care is not exclusive to members of the groups affected. The U.S. government and its agencies have likewise noted their preoccupation with problems of differential access, underutilization, adequacy, and other questions concerning the efficacy of mental health services whenever ethnic groups are involved, as they amount to de facto discrimination (Lessinger 1991:11). De facto discrimination occurs through the slippage between jural requirements of equality and the actual practices in which it is differentially implemented. Efforts toward redress and reform of this slippage have traditionally required the advocacy and activism of organized ethnic groups to mobilize state action through their self-constitution as politically significant forces.

In the mental health field, activist moments in the 1960s and 1970s fostered, among other developments, equal access to educational institutions for minorities, producing a generation of Latino mental health professionals who could assume leadership roles in the field and in its institutional politics. The convergence of Latino activism from this era with the official government concern exacted by it produced the primary normative statement on minorities' mental health care needs and rights as set forth in the 1978 Special Populations report.[1]

The report characterized Latinos as "vulnerable," as a population "at risk" in all aspects of mental health, even while recognizing the dearth of information about them. Defined as a problem for the dominant culture, Latinos were deemed to suffer the full impact of a "culture of poverty," entailing low incomes, unemployment and underemployment, undereducation, poor housing, prejudice and discrimination, and the persistence of cultural and linguistic barriers to institutional access. The low quality and quantity of

[39]

mental health services available to Latinos, the authors of the report asserted, compounded the effects of this "culture of poverty," rendering Latinos particularly susceptible to mental illness. Urban life, the youth of the population, and an extended family environment were yet other factors that predisposed Latinos to psychological and emotional stress, and thus to mental illness. The urban environment exposed Latinos to decay, poverty, and crime. Because of the predominance of young people, the bulk of the population was exposed to a "culture of poverty" at the most vulnerable stage for psychosocial development. Extended family life prevented economic progress, presumably (the assertion is not spelled out in the text) because extended families suffer a drain in material resources since they incorporate family members—the young and the old, even women—who cannot be wage earners because of their age, condition, family role, or ineligibility for the labor market (Special Populations 1978:2–3).

These are the factors that the authors of the report subsume under a "culture of poverty." But they are actually structural conditions that, strictly speaking, are not produced by and within Latino culture as such—however that should be defined—even though they become part of the sociocultural experience of the population as "immigrants" and as members of a racialized group. By the time the report was rendered, scholars had already critiqued the conceptualization of Latino social life, or that of any other group, as a "culture of poverty," noting that it amounted to a political exercise that rationalized systemic inequalities and overlooked the ways in which members of such groups strategically drew on cultural knowledge and practices in order to subsist under inimical structural conditions (Valentine 1968; Leacock 1971; Stack 1974). The report's portrayals thus constitute constructions of oppositional otherness that play upon mythical models and criteria rendering Anglo/Euro-Americans as living out their lives in ideal conditions of employment, education, housing, health, linguistic and cultural practices, and family structure and composition.

Furthermore, "culture of poverty" factors were psychologized in the report as "high stress indicators" which correlate with "personality disintegration" and "a subsequent need for treatment intervention." The report asserts:

> Beyond a doubt, [the United States] has very few programs aimed at serving the specific needs of the Spanish-speaking people. Hispanics do not receive adequate mental health services and underutilize existing services, *although a high incidence of mental problems is known to occur among this population.* Hispanics need better mental health services because, as a group, they are only partially acculturated and marginally integrated economically and, as a consequence, are subject to a number of "high stress indicators." These indicators, known to be correlated with personality disintegration and subsequent

need for treatment intervention, include (a) poor communication skills in English; (b) the poverty cycle—limited education, lower income, depressed social status, deteriorated housing and minimal political influence; (c) the survival of traits from a rural agrarian culture which are relatively ineffectual in an urban technical society; (d) the necessity for some workers for seasonal migration; (e) the stressful problem of acculturation to a society which appears prejudicial, hostile and rejecting. (Special Populations 1978:14; my emphasis)[2]

In sum, deviance from assumed dominant norms and a differential position within authorized social structures rendered Latinos psychically fragile. Within this psychologized discourse, "high stress indicators" establish relations of causality between presumed social dysfunction and the onset of mental illness to legitimize the need for incorporating cultural specificity and sensitivity in mental health treatment. Sociocultural, historical, and structural factors are thus conflated and translated into a psychological causality that becomes the rationale for policy recommendations on the delivery of public mental health services.

The authors recommended the development and implementation of "culturally-specific" models of service delivery for Latinos "which integrate the traditional values and support systems of Hispanic Americans with conventional treatment modalities such as those provided by psychiatrists and psychologists" (Special Populations 1978:15). But what the authors of the report do not note is that these "culturally-specific" models necessarily draw upon the same cultural traits and practices—"tradition," language, interactional styles—that they themselves characterize as "stress indicators" and sources of dysfunction. Their prescriptions do draw, though, upon a trend in which mental health practitioners were increasingly rediscovering "culture" as a factor in treatment.

The ambiguity with which "culture" and "cultural difference" are at once characterized as both source of dysfunction and therapeutic panacea underscores the authors' propensity for decontextualizing and typifying these constructs and refracting them through the lens of an other-dominant psychologized discourse. This was replicated in the proposals for establishing the Latino programs. A psychologized discourse contributed to the organization and reproduction of practices in which "culture" appears as a typified category rather than as a dynamic source of knowledge that underpins modes of sociocultural action.

Remarking on an apparent dearth of research on Latinos and mental health, the authors of the report did recognize contemporary research that represented Latinos in "negative" terms and compared them unfavorably to a dominant non-Latino "culture" and "values." A "mainstream" culture was again constituted as the standard and thus as the positive valence in opposi-

tion to the "minority" culture. Contemporary research, the report notes, "reveals" that

> Hispanics subsist in a "culture of poverty"; that is, they are at the bottom of the socioeconomic ladder, uneducated, unemployed, and live in substandard housing. . . . They abuse drugs and alcohol. . . . They are superstitious, unacculturated, and have clearly defined traditional and retrogressive family structures and roles. . . . Additionally, Hispanics receive mental health care of inferior quantity and quality. . . . *This could be due to the lower frequency and severity of mental illness resulting from cultural characteristics such as the extended family system, which provide protection against emotional stresses. . . .* Or it could result from their tendency to rely on faith healers (*curanderos* or *espiritistas*). . . . Or it could result from reliance upon relatives, *compadres* [co-godparents], physicians, and priests or ministers. . . . Finally, it could be that Hispanics underutilize mental health facilities because of discouraging institutional policies such as geographic isolation from centers where services are delivered, language barriers, class-bound values, and culture-bound values. . . .
>
> In terms of cross-cultural comparison, Hispanics have been found to differ from Anglos in intelligence . . . , scholastic achievement . . . , locus of control . . . , cooperational competition . . . , affective meaning of family and sex-role-related concepts . . . , responses to various clinical and personality assessment instruments . . . , and numerous sociocultural variables. (*Special Populations* 1978:22; my emphasis)

The report consequently reiterated the negative images generated by social science and medical researchers while addressing another issue: underutilization by Latinos of existing mental health programs. Yet the associations being forged in the report are enjoined in contradiction and reproduce the "culture as dysfunction/culture as cure" proposition that objectifies Latino culture. Both report and researchers thus characterize Latinos as exhibiting a "lower frequency and severity of mental illness" because of the beneficial effects of the very same "cultural characteristics" that they have redefined as stressors placing them at risk for mental illness.

The report concludes that while "Hispanics have been found to differ from the majority group in many aspects of a complex cultural spectrum," the nature of the total spectrum had not been completely elucidated, especially since the differences may be the product of "imposed etics" on the part of non-Latino researchers (Special Populations 1978:22–23). The authors urge more extensive research by "native" (Latino) researchers, because they can describe and analyze the culture with added sensitivity. The Latino mental health professionals in New York would capitalize on this recognition of inherent cultural authority.

In their concluding remarks, the report's authors identify five points that

they believe underlie their assessment of contemporary policy failings in Latino mental health issues and needs: (1) the position of Latinos as the fastest-growing minority in the United States; (2) the cultural heterogeneity of the communities that are subsumed under the term "Hispanic"; (3) the resistance to linguistic and cultural assimilation demonstrated by Latinos; (4) the preclusion of Latinos from mainstream sociocultural structures in the United States as an effect of their resistance to assimilation, which produces a systematic denial of their rights to adequate mental health care; and (5) the need for increased participation by Latinos in "shaping their own destiny." This last point was deemed the most important, one that could lead to the formulation of a national policy for improving the mental health status of Latino communities in the United States (Special Populations 1978:43). The report's final assertion thus punctuates the particularities of Latino communities in the United States, positions them as politically disadvantaged constituencies, and delivers a political appeal for increased participation to advance ethnic control over public spheres of action. In a concluding display of a discourse of entitlement that capitalizes on fundamental principles of U.S. political ideology, the authors declare that their intent is not to convey a message of ethnocentrism or isolationism but to assert foundational rights to freedom, dignity, and the pursuit of happiness (Special Populations 1978:43).

I have cited this report in detail to document the ideological context of the negotiations and to establish how the report's discursive paradoxes informed advocacy efforts in New York. A number of the core components of the discourse adopted by the programs' advocates are present there: the characterization of Latinos as a population "at risk" for mental illness; the reification of "culture"; the conflation of "cultural" features with structural conditions, and their psychologization in order to substantiate an alleged predisposition to illness; and the proposition that cultural sensitivity in mental health treatment is a solution to the problem. These were further articulated by the programs' advocates as rationales for their establishment. Woven through this discourse is the paradoxical characterization of the curative possibilities "inherent" in the "at risk" Latino culture.

The report was also instrumental in the work of my employer, the Hispanic Health Institute, which carried out the evaluation of the programs. It was one of a series of research facilities that responded to the call for intensifying research on Latino mental health issues. This call indexed a concept of culture as a factual bundle of traits to be refracted through the prism of research as the essential definition of Latino-ness, with all the referential concreteness that such a degree of typification implies. Ironically, while the pitfalls in the production of stereotypes were recognized and critiqued by the authors of the report, their own unexamined notions of culture, so

strongly conflated with class, contributed to the reproduction of negative cultural stereotypes. The Latino professionals in New York also mobilized these notions in legitimating their claims for specialized Latino programs

Finally, in addition to the need-based constitution of Latinos as a population at risk for mental illness, the Latino professionals based their demands on a number of other factors, including national demographics, cultural and linguistic difference, a presumed history of nonassimilation, and the principle of equal participation authorized by the national political order. These arguments appealed, on the one hand, to the therapeutic worldview specific to the mental health profession, while, on the other, they mobilized a basic political discourse of entitlement, civic inclusion, and participation.

The Actors Involved

The Congress for Hispanic Mental Health (CHMH), an organization of Latino mental health professionals and paraprofessionals, was founded in New York City in the 1980s. The CHMH's core membership requirement was a commitment to sustaining an active involvement in the field of mental health with special concern for the Latino community. The CHMH constituted a special interest group, one of many such local voluntary associations that have proliferated among Latino professional and occupational groups in New York City. The organization coalesced around a group of Latino leaders who were deemed key personnel in organizing and mobilizing the group as a body; most or all of them were psychiatrists and psychologists in private practice who occupied upper-level positions in the city's mental health care facilities.

Anyone could be a member of the CHMH so long as he or she was committed to supporting Latino interests. CHMH regulations defined a general member as a person of "Hispanic background" holding a graduate degree in any of the recognized mental health professions—psychiatry, psychology, social work, or psychiatric nursing—or a bachelor's degree where acceptable for entry-level professional practice in the mental health field. Affiliate members were Latinos working in other than a traditional mental health discipline, or non-Latinos with graduate degrees in a mental health discipline who were interested in Latino mental health issues. Latinos who held bachelor's degrees in other fields but were employed in mental health could also become affiliate members, as could Latino and non-Latino professionals in the law, nonpsychiatric medicine, or government service with an interest in Latino mental health issues, advocacy, or research. Student members were not required to be Latinos, but only had to be pursuing a graduate degree in a mental health discipline or a bachelor's degree for

entry-level practice in mental health. Finally, honorary membership (which could be awarded only by the CHMH's board of directors) was available to any person in any discipline who made an outstanding contribution to the mental health service delivery system for Latino communities in the greater New York City area.

Membership in the CHMH was thus based only partially on ethnicity, and even that criterion was an ambiguous one, since the qualifier "Hispanic background" was not defined; in practice it was a function mostly of self-ascription. Those CHMH members with whom I worked included all kinds of Latinos: newly arrived immigrants, first- and second-generation Latinos, and those who had come to the United States for their education and stayed to practice in the mental health field. They claimed origins in many different Spanish-speaking countries, and exhibited a wide range of language competence and preference as well as a variety of racial mixes and class status. Their diversity did not preclude the adoption of an ethnic identity produced in the host country rather than forged through a more strictly defined commonality of circumstances. The term "Hispanic background" served a paradigmatic strategy of contrast specifying non-Anglo origin, and indicated a shared stance of political activism (Padilla 1985). Gathered under this umbrella term, mental health practitioners from a variety of backgrounds could capitalize on the existing ideological order and mobilize to advocate for changes in the allocation of material and symbolic resources to benefit all the Latino communities in New York City. The virtues of the designation "Hispanic background" thus lay in its very ambiguity.

Another difference among members revolved around the power to participate in the election process and occupy leadership positions, prerogatives that were reserved for general members. Barred from this category, non-Latinos were thus excluded from voting or holding office, as were Latinos in disciplines other than the traditional mental health ones and members who did not hold the proper academic credentials for their occupational field. The distinction between "entry level mental health positions" and "entry level professional practice" seemed to me ambiguous, though it supposedly reflected one's academic training: a psychology degree as opposed to a general nursing degree, for example. CHMH membership was thus stratified, with power determined by one's professional status in the field of mental health as measured by educational and occupational credentials, understood to represent knowledge.

The CHMH's organizational focus on issues of Latino mental health was concentrated on political advocacy in executive, administrative, and legislative forums; although its leadership incorporated research and peer training among its strategies, these were secondary, or at least somewhat less visible, pursuits. CHMH leaders developed mental health policy platforms and lob-

bied for them among candidates for political office in the city and the state, supported high-level Latino appointments to city and state agencies, and proposed legislation. They also advocated for recruitment of Latino employees in public agencies, advised these agencies on Latino needs, and mobilized to provide specialized—that is, "ethnic"—crisis intervention when public resources were strained.[3] Much of this work, of course, was directed toward the establishment of specialized services for Latinos.

Difference was thus the underlying principle that governed CHMH public activities: it was codified in such phrases as "Hispanic concerns," "Hispanic mental health issues," and "Hispanic interests" to underscore a preoccupation with access to public mental health services, as well as the quality of those services. These concerns responded to perceptions that Latinos literally could not understand medical practices dealing mostly with nonphysiological pathology, in which diagnosis and treatment are language-dependent. Underlying this perception was an ingrained Cartesian belief holding that diseased organs and broken bones are objectively perceptible and treatable in their sheer materiality, but the workings of the mind and the emotions are best made intelligible when expressed through language. CHMH leaders maintained that the linguistic and cultural barriers affecting Latino mental patients also precluded their understanding and complying with prescribed treatment, thus rendering inefficacious, in the curative terms that inform psychiatric ideology, any efforts to serve the Latino patient population. Compounding the problem were the facts of migration and otherness that they believed negatively determined the Latino experience.

It should be evident that this ideological framework drew upon and articulated with the portrayal of Latinos in the report of the Special Populations panel. Indeed, in their conversations with me, CHMH leaders repeatedly referred to the report as legitimating the representations they were deploying in their own organizational efforts. The assertions about Latino identity and "culture" perpetuated in the report were transformed into self-validating rationales that took on the guise of a particular logic of entitlement to support their case.

To reiterate, the leaders capitalized on presumed facts of absolute linguistic and cultural difference. They described the alleged high incidence of mental illness among Latinos as a problem for both the dominant host culture and Latinos themselves. They advocated for consideration of cultural and linguistic difference in the psychiatric assessment and treatment of Latino patients as imperative for improving the quality of mental health programs. Finally, they depicted migration and cultural difference as circumstances with definitive pathological consequences, as "stress indicators" that at a minimum aggravated and at worst caused mental illness among Latinos. This discourse framed the strategies of entitlement that CHMH

leaders deployed in their advocacy efforts with city and state mental health bureaucracies and that permeated all of the organization's activities.

The CHMH mounted major efforts to deal with the two agencies that administer mental health care in the New York metropolitan area: the city's Health and Hospitals Corporation (HHC) and the New York State Office of Mental Health (OMH). The HHC oversees city hospitals and general health services, while the OMH monitors state mental health facilities, but their spheres of administrative action overlap. Most important, the state agency provides funding for the city's mental health programs, and has the power to monitor shifts in the city's funding priorities if any change is not approved beforehand. In this sense, the relationship between the two is somewhat stratified and prone to contestation and negotiation.

The HHC was initially created in 1969 by the state as a public benefit corporation to organize and administer the finances of the city's public hospital facilities. The tradition of public hospital care in New York City dates to 1736. Ever since then the City Charter has guaranteed public health care to all residents regardless of their capacity to pay (Kramer 1977:55). Predictably, ethno-racial "minorities" currently make up a large proportion of the city hospitals' clients. OMH is charged with assuring the availability of high-quality care to all state residents through its state mental health facilities, by funding mental health services operated by municipal governments, and by planning and overseeing the finances of all mental health programs in the state (Governor's Advisory Committee for Hispanic Affairs n.d.).

The Negotiations

Dr. Ramírez, a Latino psychiatrist and first president of the CHMH, reconstructed the process for different members of the evaluation team, including me, in a series of interviews and conversations over the years. In 1984, when the CHMH was newly founded, its leaders first proposed the establishment of a bilingual, bicultural psychiatric program for the city's Latino population; but they were targeting a city hospital, not a state facility. With the support of an HHC vice president (who happened to be one of the city's most prominent Latino psychiatrists), the idea was presented to the OMH commissioner, who referred the proposal to OMH's New York City regional office; neither the OMH commissioner nor OMH's regional director was Latino.

This period represented CHMH's first major advocacy effort with OMH, and the Latino programs were but one item in an agenda that included a wide array of Latino mental health projects. Upon receiving this agenda, the OMH regional director requested a private meeting with Dr. Ramírez

[47]

to discuss the establishment of a bilingual, bicultural program. It was then that the issue of segregation was first raised—one that would beleaguer the programs throughout their establishment and institutionalization. The regional director maintained that such specialized programs explicitly violated a core clinical and institutional goal in mental health treatment: the assimilation of ethnic mental patients into the dominant culture. Dr. Ramírez argued that his goal was to provide medical services that were greatly needed by the city's Latinos, an objective that did not in itself preclude assimilation. OMH committed "to go halfway" if city officials did likewise, thus requiring CHMH to engage in further negotiations. But when CHMH presented its extensive agenda to the city's commissioner of mental health, all of the issues "became diluted," as Dr. Ramírez expressed it, which he characterized as "a major strategical mistake" on the part of CHMH. This seemed to be the outcome of an advocacy agenda whose very ambitiousness made it hard to implement.

The segregation issue reemerged two years later, when grassroots efforts to implement specialized services for Latinos, which had been initiated independently at Plymouth Psychiatric Center (located outside New York City) in 1982, became public. These efforts came about through the endeavors of a Latina social worker who believed that language barriers were detrimental to the quality of institutional life for Plymouth's Latino patients. She organized informal therapy and activity groups, in which Latino patients were able to speak Spanish among themselves and with staff, discuss current events from Latino newspapers, listen to Latino music, and occasionally even enjoy Latino food. Other staff at the facility became invested in generating more specialized services for their Latino patients, and more groups were organized for them.

Although Plymouth is a state mental health facility under OMH jurisdiction, neither the OMH central office in Albany nor the regional office in New York City was aware that its staff were engaged in creating local institutional conditions that would culminate in the establishment of a bilingual, bicultural program for Latino patients. Some officials at the central office later claimed that it was only through newspaper articles that they heard of these efforts. The agency had to disclaim official support for the incipient program at Plymouth when a sudden spurt of publicity provoked controversy within the central office over the thought of a program for Latinos emerging, unauthorized, in their midst. Even more hostility and resistance were triggered when Plymouth's Latino staff officially requested support from upper-level administrators at the facility for the institutionalization of their heretofore informal program.

An official at the OMH central office who was sympathetic to the concept of ethnically sensitive care described the reaction of his colleagues as "con-

sternation": the idea of "Hispanic mental care," they maintained, was "a bunch of bullshit." The schism between sympathizers and detractors was not necessarily drawn along ethnic lines. Latino staff at OMH argued that the provision of a specialized program for Latinos would actually result in the deterioration of services for them. The programs would end up under-staffed, Latino patients would be placed in physically inferior facilities, and the whole effort would constitute merely "a nice show" for politicians. In their minds, separation engendered inequality, a principle arising from the history of civil rights litigation that has entered both official and popular discourse in the United States.[4] Latinos at the central office also suspected that the state would not commit resources on a long-term basis; as a result, the programs would be in an insecure financial position "when the gravy train ran out." Bureaucratic objections from "natives" thus merged ideolog-ical arguments with a pragmatic, even skeptical assessment of state political interests and actions.

Another focus of contention originated in press reports that a local NAACP chapter had charged that the program for Hispanics was segrega-tionist. OMH's concern extended to the possibility that the agency could be "legally exposed" if these charges generated legal action by Latino interest groups. Conversely, the programs could be interpreted as an instance of ethnic favoritism, raising the opposite possibility that other ethnic groups would institute legal action. Interethnic friction and competition for state resources were clearly threatening specters.

A high-level official at the OMH central office later attributed the success of Plymouth staff in implementing their program to the fact that they "moved slowly and small": the programmatic changes they instituted did not entail major shifts in institutional resources and priorities. Changes were carried out incrementally so that "staff at the different levels of the ad-ministrative hierarchy did not feel alienated." Plymouth staff were able to articulate a rationale for the changes by equating a language barrier to inad-equacy of institutional care. The modesty of their efforts allowed them bet-ter control over institutional outcomes, as the success of their innovations was "proven" by measuring behavioral improvement in the small and famil-iar group of patients they worked with.

The strategies that Plymouth staff were deploying were obviously similar to those that the CHMH was developing. Both Plymouth staff and CHMH leaders based their arguments in part on the strategy of representing lin-guistic and cultural barriers as impediments to adequate mental health care for Hispanics, and thus as a violation of the principle of equality in the de-livery of service. Plymouth staff were in a position to substantiate these ar-guments by documenting them through "successful" clinical outcomes, that is, by using their patients' medical histories to show "progress" as indicated

by a reduction in medication, increased participation in institutional activities, and/or an increased patient discharge rate—the best index possible. These outcome-oriented success narratives were further legitimized in terms of bureaucratic and medical ideologies heavily invested in the "curative" effect of their institutional practices, as well as an efficiency model used in "processing" patients through the system.

Two additional contextual factors favored Plymouth staff's efforts. Plymouth's upper-level administrators were known for their "open door" policy: they encouraged staff at all levels to discuss issues with hospital executives and offer suggestions for improving services. Local institutional support among upper-level administrators contributed to legitimizing the evolving efforts of Latino staff to formalize their endeavor and supported their claims regarding the need for the program.

In addition, Plymouth served a high proportion of Latino patients, its catchment area included numerous Latino communities, and it had many Latinos on staff. Prior to the widespread trend toward deinstitutionalization in the 1970s, Plymouth had been the largest psychiatric care facility in the nation. Beginning in the 1930s, immigrant Latinos flocked to it to avail themselves of work opportunities in lower-level, nonprofessional positions. Latino residents of the area still constituted a labor pool as well as a patient pool for Plymouth.[5] Latinos were the predominant ethnic presence at Plymouth and in the community—a circumstance that would distinguish it from the other two programs, which were sited in facilities with somewhat more heterogeneous ethno-racial staff and patient populations. The Plymouth program did not have to contend to the degree that the other two did with the presence of patients from other groups who could equally claim specialized needs. It was thus easier for Plymouth staff to justify the institutionalization of a Latino program.

The high-level OMH official cited earlier also articulated the bureaucratic ideology that governed the implementation of institutional changes at OMH: "good" ideas may be conceptually validated on their "scientific merits" and their "humanistic qualities," but their implementation is another matter because it requires assessing their consequences in the realms of politics, economics, and vested institutional concerns. Central to the balance of interests is a win-lose proposition: who will win and who will lose as a result of the implementation of a "good" idea must always be kept in mind. Plymouth staff had started cautiously, proved the therapeutic possibilities, and garnered internal institutional support to demonstrate the potential of a bilingual, bicultural program. The question remained whether the Plymouth experience could be writ large in the broader realm of vested interests in state policy. In the realpolitik of bureaucratic ideology, the legitimacy of establishing specialized Latino programs had to be "sold"—as Dr.

Ramírez, the CHMH leadership, and other sympathizers soon realized—in political and practical terms as a cost-effective and superior service. Their arguments for establishing the programs could not succeed solely on their merits as a specialized service that would fulfill a particular group's medical needs, and even less as a request from an organization of ethnic professionals advocating for their own people; the arguments also had to be "pragmatic" in political and administrative terms.

In the meantime, OMH had rejected Plymouth's request for the institutionalization of its program. In the view of the sympathetic official at OMH's central office, staff at Plymouth were being asked "to stop doing whatever it was they were doing" as a result of considerable political pressure being brought to bear through the OMH hierarchy. An OMH affirmative action official tried to persuade him that what was taking place at Plymouth was clearly discriminatory; while he disagreed, it seemed apparent that "bureaucratic realities" had finally overcome the Plymouth program, and with it the idea of specialized Latino programs.

Plymouth staff, however, had appealed to CHMH for support, thus resurrecting among its leadership the issue of culturally sensitive mental health care and the possibility of establishing bilingual, bicultural psychiatric programs. It was this moment of convergence that participants would later identify as the "real" initial round in the struggle that characterized the negotiations.

Although the chronology and details of events were somewhat unclear by the time I began my fieldwork, the CHMH started by mobilizing strategies of advocacy in other forums. "Talking about the problem"—that is, negotiating the establishment of the programs—went on between CHMH leaders and officials from the Governor's Committee for Hispanic Affairs and its counterpart in the New York City mayor's office. A major achievement at this stage was garnering the support of African Americans on OMH's Minority Advisory Committee, as well as a public pronouncement by the NAACP's regional director that the concept of culturally sensitive care was neither segregationist nor discriminatory. These manifestations of interethnic support fortified CHMH's efforts, and thus the negotiations, since both non-Latino administrators and Latino leaders considered African Americans the only other minority in the city with the visibility, sense of marginalized participation, and political clout to forestall CHMH's efforts.

Significantly, CHMH leaders focused their energies on minimizing the aura of distinction and otherness—a major cause of bureaucratic unease— that the establishment of the programs entailed. They strategically emphasized language difference; that is, they represented culturally sensitive care as hinging mainly on the use of fully bilingual staff in the programs. The "cultural" issue was deemphasized to avoid the delicate problems of distin-

guishing conceptually and practically between language and culture, defining Latino-ness, and discerning subtle cultural differences across a multinational Latino population. The leaders also thus avoided the more general issues of establishing the boundaries of ethnic identity and exploring the problematic relationship between cultural difference and universalistic medical ideologies and practices. This last was the most complex issue that had to be "solved." Ultimately it was addressed through the programmatic goal of developing culturally sensitive modalities of psychiatric care in the programs themselves. Since acculturating patients into the dominant culture is a major institutional goal in the treatment of ethnic minorities, any appearance that the programs could contribute to the maintenance of cultural separatism would have alarmed public officials, and so had to be avoided. Finally, concerns about cost-effectiveness were allayed by stressing that both the state and city systems already had on staff bilingual Latino mental health practitioners who could be recruited to work in the programs.

CHMH leaders also capitalized on the ambiguities surrounding language. In "talking about the problem," they stressed the apparently organic nature of language acquisition. That is, they "naturalized" competence in Spanish as innate to Latino patients (with ramifications that I explore further in subsequent chapters). They exploited popular notions about the process as being the "natural" outcome of being born in a particular culture, a matter over which no individual can exert control. Learning and using a second language, they implied, pertain to culture and are thus the product of a degree of volition available to the sane but not necessarily to the mentally ill.[6] The programs, CHMH leaders insisted, would be identical to others except that they would be bilingual.

At an early point in the negotiations, as part of their "selling strategy" CHMH leaders suggested establishing a demonstration project with an evaluation component, which was rationalized as a way to substantiate the project's worth in political and bureaucratic terms. As Dr. Ramírez would later point out, "[State government officials] want[ed] to hear this kind of thing."

What government officials at OMH wanted to hear was predicated on their perceptions of the programs as a controversial proposition contrary to an institutional policy of ensuring equality through the desegregation of mental health services. The fact of language difference, however, made notions of "equality" ambiguous. Because CHMH leaders had made the case, on institutional and medical grounds, that the language barrier between Latinos and mental health personnel impinged on issues of access to mental health services and quality of care, state officials were caught up in the contradictions that surround equality as an administrative, legal, and practical standard.

Institutional equality dictates that the same kinds of services be offered to all populations, thus equating social, political, and cultural equality with uniformity of access to institutional resources. In this sense, providing bilingual, bicultural services to Latinos but not to other groups could be construed as discriminatory. Conversely, though, the practical consequences of *not* treating Latinos—a politically significant community in the state and in the city—in their native language exposed the agency to charges of limiting their access to efficacious medical and institutional resources. Bureaucrats were faced with mental health practitioners claiming on the basis of both cultural and occupational knowledge that the care being provided was deficient. Their charges of de facto discrimination had serious political and legal consequences for OMH, coming as they did from an organized advocacy group of Latinos who were constituting themselves as part of a larger demographic and political force. In this way CHMH leaders exploited the slippage intrinsic to discourses about equality in the United States.

"Culture" as Cure: Program Evaluation

Given the need to justify the programs to public officials preoccupied with political and jural concerns and invested in the agendas of their institutional culture, CHMH leaders were compelled to propose the evaluation of the programs. Assessing their worth would legitimate the institutionalization of culturally sensitive care. The questions of what and how to evaluate were articulated by the outcome-governed ethos of bureaucratic and medical ideologies but also, like the programs themselves, capitalized on cultural and linguistic difference.

Evaluation in this context is predicated on the belief that social programs have ameliorating effects on problematic aspects of social life in complex modern societies. It involves the production of knowledge that can be applied toward improving the social programs on which it is brought to bear. But evaluation is also embedded in the political world of special interests and the promotion of ideologies that inspire those who attempt to affect the policies of any public program. The strongly political purposes that surround evaluation are a complicating factor for anyone who expects it to be an exercise in scientific objectivity (Cook and Shadish 1986:197–98).

According to Dr. Ramírez, when negotiating the terms of the evaluation itself, CHMH resisted officials' efforts to devise evaluation components that would make the programs "complicated." This was consonant with CHMH's strategies in representing the programs as a cost-effective and manageable proposition that would be identical to any other inpatient men-

tal health program, except for employing Spanish-speaking staff. CHMH leaders drafted their own proposals with arguments that explicitly drew from and reiterated the constructs formulated in the presidential report, invoking demographic factors, risk, resistance to assimilation, the dearth of services, resource underutilization, and the psychologization of "culture" as both source of dysfunction and therapeutic panacea. The historic endurance of Latino cultural and linguistic difference in the United States was also invoked—in paradoxically ahistorical terms, since it is projected into the future as an intrinsic, ineradicable cultural trait that must be dealt with programmatically through mental health ministrations.

By the spring of 1987, CHMH leaders had produced a series of proposals directed to the establishment of two bilingual, bicultural Spanish-language inpatient psychiatric units with an evaluation component.[7] The proposal that eventually prevailed began by noting that the "fair" delivery of mental health services is preconditioned on both a shared language and sensitivity to cultural issues. The presumed lack of English competence among Latinos is characterized as an aggravating factor in the strain of mental illness, and thus analogous to a clinical condition. Linguistic difference, CHMH leaders contended, constitutes Latinos as a "special needs" group—giving credence to Flores and Yúdice's (1990) critique that Latino communities are constituted mostly in terms of needs assessment.[8] Language difference thus requires the establishment of a specialized ("language-syntonic") program to counter the effects of cultural and linguistic estrangement produced and compounded by migration.

The ideological core of the CHMH proposal articulated cultural difference in medicalized terms: "Using the traditional medical model, patients are to be grouped around the issues of language and communication so relevant to psychiatry in the same manner that patients are grouped around specialized staff and services for the purposes of emergency care, obstetrical needs, gastrointestinal diseases, pediatrics, geriatrics, etc." Cultural and linguistic differences were thus infused with an aura of alienation and pathology, incorporated into the medical model, and reconstructed as a medicalized domain of treatment.

The proposal's authors shared the caution that surrounded the political maneuvering in the negotiations; they insisted that they were contemplating the provision not of preferential services but "of regular and standard psychiatric services in an atmosphere which is propitious for optimal communication." Relying on then-current clinical interpretations of language use, they stressed the primary role of Spanish in therapeutic interventions even among bilinguals by promoting the notion that bilinguals master their host language for "instrumental" purposes but resort to the native language for "expressive" purposes.[9] Since linguistic "expressiveness" is essential in

psychiatry and psychology to access mental processes, therapy was gravely hampered by linguistic dissimilarity between therapist and patient even among bilinguals. This notion of linguistic "regression" had the practical effect of making the programs appropriate for a broader spectrum of Latino patients, bilingual as well as monolingual.

The proposal explicitly incorporated "cultural sensitivity" as a major element in the programs' design, articulated in terms of empathy in the "use of cultural referents in the provision of services" for their assumed therapeutic value: "By placing the patient in a familiar therapeutic milieu, his [sic] contact with reality is facilitated and enhanced." The proposal identified the referential contents of cultural sensitivity as art, "folk" food, "tradition," and alternative therapeutic approaches that the drafters characterize as "culture-bound" because they are "a reflection" of a patient's culture.

The evaluation component devised in the proposal focuses on assessing quality of care by equating the assumed "fact" of linguistic and cultural difference with the deprivation of adequate services—the same principle that underpinned the arguments for establishing the programs. The drafters proposed an evaluation design organized into the three-stage assessment that I have already described, in which programmatic goals were replicated in a design that addressed three parallel processual aspects of the programs' institutionalization.

CHMH was not directly engaged in the evaluation itself: once the programs were established, its advocacy role had been fulfilled. Some CHMH leaders, notably those who had spearheaded the efforts to establish the programs, were nevertheless recruited to sit on the advisory boards that were created for each; others were appointed to positions in the programs themselves. These mental health professionals continued to exert authority over the implementation of the programs as members of these bodies. They also constituted an "informal" source of information, consultation, and political leverage for the evaluation, and were often called upon to mediate problems that emerged in the programs. Their presence further contributed to perpetuating the representations deployed during the negotiations.

The Hispanic Health Institute

The Hispanic Health Institute (HHI) was the organization contracted to evaluate the psychiatric programs.[10] Though it slightly preceded the panel's report to the president's commission, its establishment in 1977 responded to the same atmosphere of concern and ethno-racial activism that led to the appointment of the commission and the production of the report. It was one of a series of research institutes that sprouted around the nation; its

mission was to implement the report's call for research. The HHI was mostly staffed by psychologists and sociologists, whose orientations greatly influenced its work through the application of these disciplinary frames of interpretation.

The institute's specific goals were explicitly directed toward "policy-relevant" research on the epidemiology of mental health and on clinical services, with a focus on the mental health problems of Latinos in the United States and in Puerto Rico. At the time of the evaluation, it had developed a conceptual framework structured along a model course of mental illness and therapeutic treatment that organized its research into five priority areas: the cultural factors and conditions involved in the emergence of mental health problems; the utilization of mental health facilities and processes of mental health assessment; the development, assessment, and study of culturally sensitive therapeutic modalities; patient compliance issues; and patient post-treatment adjustment. This framework itself reflected the strong clinical orientation of HHI research as well as the similarities between its own research agenda and the programmatic goals proposed for the Latino programs.

Cultural sensitivity was also an explicit core component of HHI's research efforts and products. The concept, staff at the institute would privately admit, was not unambiguous. HHI staff drew upon a working definition of cultural sensitivity that, from an anthropological perspective, gave their work a strong functionalist cast:

> We do not begin with an *a priori* definition of what constitutes culturally sensitive mental health care; rather, we examine how the concept has been used by mental health practitioners and researchers in their work with Hispanics. In doing so, we argue that there are three meanings. First, rendering the treatment more accessible to Hispanic clients by taking into account their cultural characteristics. Second, selecting or altering an available therapeutic modality according to features of Hispanic culture. Third, extracting elements from Hispanic culture and using them as a treatment modality. (Costantino, Malgady, and Rogler 1985:2)

Accessibility of service could be contingent on the use of bilingual, bicultural staff or the use of translators; more vaguely, it hinged on incorporating into the service cultural elements that "are there" (Costantino, Malgady, and Rogler 1985:3–4). For example, one of the Latino programs added an outpatient clinic that accommodated walk-in visits. Under the first of these "meanings" of cultural sensitivity, this would be rationalized as a "recognized" cultural idiosyncrasy of Latino patients because Latinos, being crisis-rather than prevention-oriented, are not inclined to make medical appoint-

ments or keep to an appointment schedule. Thus the necessity for a walk-in policy.

Altering existing treatment modalities to render them culturally sensitive, the second definition, postulated an isomorphic, mirrorlike relationship between treatment and the patient's assumed cultural "characteristics" (Costantino, Malgady, and Rogler 1985:8). For example, HHI researchers urged the acknowledgment of folk beliefs—in *espiritismo, santería,* or *brujería* (witchcraft)—and their integration into treatment modalities under the control of the therapist.

The third "meaning" of cultural sensitivity required the "extraction" of cultural elements for use as a treatment modality; it was best exemplified in the Latino programs by the effort to ethnicize time and space, as I describe in the next chapter. Staff at the programs strongly believed in the therapeutic effect on the patient of immersion in a total environment (cf. Goffman 1961). Creating an ethnicized milieu through the use of Latino art, music, food, activities, and celebrations, it followed, would *automatically* provide a culturally sensitive context in which the application of traditional therapy would become more efficacious for Latino patients.

Thus the three "meanings" accorded to the notion of cultural sensitivity underscore how the concept of culture as such was articulated as a reservoir of content that is drawn upon to be inserted into another domain comprehended as cultureless, universal, and objective. Treatment therapies, rather than being constituted as cultural relationships structured through medical and institutional discourses, ideologies, and practices, were viewed as value-free instrumental entities.

Despite their adoption of these definitions in attempting to systematize the concept of culturally sensitive care, HHI staff often expressed to me their concern with the ambiguity of the concept. The application of anthropological methodologies and principles to the evaluation of the Latino programs represented an innovation in HHI's work intended to enhance and transcend its reliance on psychological and sociological frames of understanding. This became particularly important since these functionalist definitions of cultural sensitivity equally informed the implementation of the programs.

In the context of HHI's clinically directed work, the evaluation of these three programs represented a conceptual shift of focus from the psychiatric to the cultural. But in practice it was still framed and strongly informed by a clinical orientation. Once the psychiatric was construed as an objective, value-free, decultured context, the cultural then became the variable object of inquiry to be identified, extracted, and applied in the Latino programs for its etiological and therapeutic value.

[3]

Clinical Topographies

The first of the Latino programs I visited was Plymouth, in June 1989, when I was introduced to program staff as a new member of the evaluation team by one of our research assistants; I thus entered the field at the pioneer site in developing a Latino-inflected mental health program. My most intensive previous experience with closed (or total) institutions had been in prisons, during the years I spent practicing public interest law and doing prison reform work. Because many of my clients alleged mental illness (most of which remained unproven, although some was diagnosed and legitimated), I had become familiar with clinical spaces, ideologies, discourses, and practices both inside and outside prisons, including the totalizing aspects of psychiatric institutions, and thus gained a comparative perspective on the varieties of experience such institutions can produce.

It has become a social science truism that total institutions forge particular forms of social interactions and an encompassing culture that set them off as a special class among sociocultural domains. Goffman's (1961) classic collection of essays on the social situation created by total institutions locates their essential character in the destruction of the boundaries that we commonly construct between everyday activities in terms of space, time, authority, and purpose (1961:6). He argues that life in total institutions is subject to certain constraints: activities are tightly scheduled; daily life is shared with a fixed group of people whose identities have been formally categorized; authority is localized and hierarchical; and activities and interactions are regulated for the sake of surveillance and management. Everything is designed to deculturize patients and induct them into an institu-

tional way of life. Staff attempt to efface signs of the outside world for a series of ideological and utilitarian purposes; in the case of psychiatric institutions, clinical rationales are advanced to legitimate this effacement.

Goffman's discussions of total institutions are framed, for analytical purposes, in the Weberian mode of ideal types; I cite them in this spirit. In practice, attempts to efface the outside world are never wholly successful. They operate at various levels of consciousness on the part of gate-keepers and inmates alike. This ambiguity reflects the prevalent social situation, in which dominant practices and discourses coexist alongside other subordinate ones (de Certeau 1984), and implicates Bourdieu's notion of institutions as durable sets of social relations endowing individuals with power (1977, 1990). In de Certeau's and Bourdieu's senses, institutions become prime sites of contestation. Challenges to institutional power are often embodied in reform movements that constitute the mentally ill, prisoners, students, and other occupants of total institutions as legal agents in order to transgress institutional totality. But by constituting these groups as legal subjects, reform has the paradoxical effect of masking the reconstitution of the totality of their situation. What appear as reforming breaches of totality are still mediated through relations of authority that determine the actual institutional experience for both staff and inmates. This mediation contributes to the reproduction of ever more subtle forms of totality—often more diffusely located—rather than rupturing it.

An example is the purposeful "ethnicization" of institutional times and spaces in the Latino programs, by which their staff, acting on the basis of recognized and self-proclaimed professional and cultural authority, inserted elements of their choice from the outside ("ethnic") world into the clinical setting for therapeutic purposes. The intention of breaching totality, reallocating resources, and reconstituting patients as cultural agents was rendered ambiguous and multivalent. The "ethnicization" pursued in the programs was not just the product of a desire to ease institutional life for Latino patients; it emanated from an explicitly clinical agenda. For Latino staff, it was a defining activity for developing culturally sensitive modalities psychiatric of care.

According to the program proposal, the "ethnicization" of institutional times and spaces in the Latino programs involved the alteration of their clinical ambience to provide a culturally "empathetic" environment for Latino patients. Program staff spoke of this process in terms of "milieu therapy," stressing the totalizing therapeutic effects that cultural elements were expected to exert over patients. Milieu therapy indexes how each interaction, event, and process within the programs' clinical spaces is expected to affect the condition and course of each patient's mental illness. Program staff held to an explicit therapeutic goal, however ideal—to cure, or at least

alleviate, psychopathy—even while recognizing that this was not their sole purpose, because the programs were also demonstration projects with strong political overtones.

Ethnicizing the clinical environment at the programs was thus designed to articulate with political, institutional, and medical "curative" models. From a medical perspective, staff talked about ethnicizing their environment as an interim goal whose "real" purpose was to facilitate the implementation of culturally sensitive modalities of care. It was also necessary to achieve high rates of discharge in order to validate the programs, since institutional bureaucracies are directed toward discharge rates as a means of documenting the elusive goal of "treating" patients toward health. This index of success is necessary for practitioners' self-validation; lack of some visible measure of success would be politically unacceptable in public mental health care. "Cure" thus remains a core discursive component of institutional culture, characterizing a patient's institutional life as a transformative process.

The clinical spaces in which the Latino programs were located were culturally specific therapeutic enclaves, a product of a Western medical ideology of care and its attendant practices. Staff, however, constituted these clinical settings not as a cultural or an ideological domain, but as a decultured space for objective clinical undertakings legitimated by the highly rationalized norms of psychiatric practice. They saw themselves as inserting what they understood to be core elements of Latino culture into this presumably blank, cultureless space in order to advance the goal of culturally sensitive psychiatric care.

Actually, the organization of space, time, and so on was hardly dissimilar to that in other psychiatric wards, despite the self-conscious attempts to ethnicize the environment and alter modalities of treatment. But these attempts actually did create, as staff and patients would express it, a "tone" of communality that they recognized and learned to value—a perceived ethnic ambience. These attempts at ethnicization also helped garner public acknowledgment of the programs' special character.

Itemizing Culture

Ambience was represented in evaluation reports as a checklist of material signs and organizational features that, in keeping with the progression established for the programs, were to be gradually achieved in their evolution toward culturally sensitive care. For the purpose of recording and reporting "progress," the evaluation team's research assistants were sent on forays to confirm that all the components of ambiance, as embodied in the list, were

in place, even though many of the items were easily perceptible. The inventory included decor, artwork, plants, displays, food, signs in Spanish, Spanish media, outings to Latino-related events, and visits by Latino "cultural" groups. All of these were understood as vehicles subject to transformation into codified aspects of Latino ethnicity, and thus held potential therapeutic power.

Curiously, the checklist also included two other elements—the provision of medication forms in Spanish and "cultural sensitivity" training for program staff—as part of the programs' "ambience." Cultural sensitivity training was a rather ambiguous requirement which the programs were to grapple with throughout their existence as demonstration projects. It aptly crystallized the objectified notion of culture that was being applied in the programs: that is, "natives" had to be trained in the "native culture" in order to become culturally sensitive.

A dose of cultural reflexivity was certainly desirable, but the few instances in which any of the programs attempted to implement the mandate proved that staff were still addressing culture only in its most concrete forms. For example, one of the programs scheduled a conference by a noted Puerto Rican anthropologist in order to fulfill this requirement. Already considered quite conservative in Puerto Rico at the time, the anthropologist embarked on a rote, objectified account of Puerto Rican culture that avoided its contemporary complexities and left unaddressed the cultural production of the diasporic Latino community. Another cultural sensitivity training session was led by a psychologist who proceeded to characterize Latino culture in very stereotypical terms, correlating cultural "features" with pathological conditions and stressing their avowedly psychogenic nature.[1] "Latino culture" was thus located as a concrete knowledge domain and articulated paradoxically as dysfunctional. I sometimes suspected that the very failure to fully implement the training mandate documented how counterintuitive it was.

Medication forms were given to patients upon discharge to instruct them about their prescriptions, including schedule of administration and side effects, as well as individual requirements for outpatient care—where, when, and to whom to appeal for therapy. Some programs managed to implement the requirement for supplying forms in Spanish, but it became a subject of amusement among research assistants who discovered that some of the programs already had translated medication forms on hand because of a longstanding city requirement, but had not used them because they thought of the programs as special efforts to incorporate "culture" into their practices. In the rarefied context in which culture was being addressed, the existing forms did not appear "special" enough.

The itemization of culture had been suggested in the programs' proposal

before I joined the evaluation team. It was at first unclear to me to what extent the inclusion of Spanish medical forms and sensitivity training was dictated by expediency on the one hand or their particular value on the other. In working with program staff, I realized, though, that their inclusion underscored the totality with which the clinical setting was being imagined. Staff training in cultural sensitivity had the potential to standardize the desired "empathetic" behavior between patients and staff, while the use of medical forms in Spanish represented the extension of the clinical into patients' lives post-discharge.

We did not totally codify the "cultural" elements in the list; they also embodied the understanding of the Latino practitioners involved in the programs as to how ethnicity should be configured and inscribed in the institutional space. The list of elements constituted an index of the ways in which ethnicity—and "culture"—was being perceived and deployed on behalf of Latino patients by those who had been granted the authority to speak for them. The list conflated emic and etic cultural categories in an effort to deconstruct Latino culture for evaluatory and therapeutic purposes.

These issues of ambience brought to the fore the relationships involved in the deployment of cultural features to mediate representations of ethnicity. Beyond its textualization in an evaluation list, the actual creation of an ethnic environment rested mostly in the hands of program staff. The choice of symbols, the definition of "ethnic," and the cultural "content" that was to be deployed were managed by a group of people whose perceptions about ethnicity were shaped by the need to legitimate the programs. But their actions were also informed by their "folk" interpretation of what culture is supposed to be "about." The representations thus produced were both inwardly and outwardly directed: they signaled ethnic solidarity, established the programs' identity, and demarcated boundaries between these specialized programs and non-Latino ones. But they also constituted ethnic simulacra within institutional spaces that were intended to function for the patients' curative benefit and to initiate the conceptualization of culturally sensitive modalities of care.

Plymouth Psychiatric Center: The Pioneer Program

Latino staff at Plymouth were highly conscious of their pioneer standing. When they began their efforts to devise an informal Latino program in 1982, they drew upon a patient population that was predominantly elderly and highly institutionalized, men and women with few remaining ties to the outside world. These circumstances by themselves rendered their potential for discharge minimal. For these patients, the discontinuity from "normal-

ity" that mental illness represents had been transformed, through the passage of time, into existential and sociocultural continuity. It was precisely because of the time they had spent in mental institutions that Plymouth's patient population was often represented as the most typical in the three Latino programs—closest to the idealized Latino mental patient constructed by advocates for the programs in order to justify their establishment. The program's patients were consistently characterized as largely monolingual or Spanish-dominant first-generation Puerto Rican immigrants whose contact with the host culture had been curtailed by mental illness, and who had been frozen in their ethnic identity by institutional isolation. This representational strategy allowed Latino professionals at Plymouth to propose that restoring ethnicity in their patients' lives would increase their potential for discharge. Given their high degree of institutionalization, however, discharge would be nearly miraculous, and this made Plymouth a particularly apposite testing ground for the curative possibilities of cultural sensitivity.

The actual profile of the patient population at Plymouth was more nuanced, and matched only some of the idealized descriptors. Participant observation, supported by the statistics we collected, amply documented that, although the population was predominantly Puerto Rican, the majority of the patients displayed bilingual competence. Plymouth's elderly patients belonged to a generation that had experienced, over the first half of the twentieth century, a colonial history of linguistic policies imposed by the United States that fostered bilingualism on the island.[2] The patients did manifest a strong cultural identification with Puerto Rico, evidencing the endurance that cultural nationalism has consistently exerted over Puerto Rican identity as a whole, but they also had spent lengthy portions of their lives in the United States either before they were institutionalized or as the product of circular migration between island and mainland; these were not immigrants "fresh off the boat." The neatness of constructing these elderly patients as primordial types was tempting, and I myself was sometimes prone to confuse the population with the image, imagining them as a monolingual, monocultural, traditionalist cohort. Yet the gap between model and actual conditions underscored one of the crucial issues in treating ethno-racial groups through institutional means: the need to locate and historicize them, both in particular and within the context of their relations with other groups, so as to transcend reductive stereotyping.

The participants in the first informal Hispanic Social Group included Latino patients from different wards at Plymouth; they became the patient population of the two gender-segregated wards where the Latino program was first unofficially attempted in 1985. After its formal initiation as a demonstration project in 1987, a recurring challenge emerged. Labor prob-

lems hindered the implementation of the program when non-Latino staff challenged their transfer out of the newly established Latino wards. This remained one of the most intractable issues throughout the implementation of the Plymouth program.

Underlying local labor tensions, variably explicit, were the same charges of segregation, discrimination, and preferential treatment that affected the institutionalization of all three programs. Non-Latino staff who were transferred out of the wards in order to accommodate exclusively Latino staffing complained that Plymouth's administrators had imposed decisions about staff allocation and ward reorganization without due consultation or prior notice. They also expressed a proprietary interest in "their" wards: through long-term daily contact, they had become familiar with ward patients, and this in turn eased their own institutional tasks. Long-standing staff relationships on a particular ward would be similarly affected, since transfer entailed the loss of seniority and informal authority acquired through lengthy service on a single ward. Last, the program's need for bilingual staff generated suspicion and resentment that "outsiders" would be recruited.[3] Plymouth's labor problems culminated in the initiation of a union grievance procedure that wended its sticky way toward arbitration and was still unresolved at the end of the evaluation fieldwork.[4]

The availability of official union action led non-Latinos at Plymouth to express their objections to the program in a formal discourse of labor rights rather than in overt but informal charges of interethnic competition, discrimination, racism, and vitiated political advancement that these objections took in the other two programs, where no official labor action was ever taken. The union option thus minimized the sometimes blatant expressions of ethnic conflict found at Jefferson and at Northern, although it did not completely preclude them.[5] The translation of interethnic political concerns into a highly localized labor dispute transformed a local process of cultural and political displacement into one of occupational displacement, amenable to management through institutional labor resources accessible to all Plymouth staff. A certain degree of apparent harmony was thus maintained, but it masked discriminatory stances and pronouncements—or at least ensured their public invisibility.

In spite of these problems, the initiation of a Hispanic day program in 1986 was rather more successful—and less controversial—than the establishment of the original wards, because it did not entail staff relocation but was created "from scratch" and staffed by those who worked on the Hispanic wards.[6] With the official establishment of the Latino programs in 1987, the two inpatient wards and the day program constituted the bilingual, bicultural psychiatric program at Plymouth. Shortly after, the patients in each of the two gender-specific wards were united in a single coed ward.

The administrative decision to unify the wards was represented as the product of practical considerations: it would minimize the controversy surrounding transfers and reduce staffing requirements. There was another strategic dimension: the decision allowed staff to refine the criteria of patient eligibility and winnow out the oldest, most dysfunctional patients. Eligibility was not predicated solely upon language competence (the standard remained Spanish monolingualism, in consonance with the ideal patient "type"). The patients selected were required to be high-functioning, exhibit potential for discharge, offer no security risks, and be "volunteers": that is, patients had to express their willingness to participate in the program, as this constitutes in psychiatric practice a sign of "normality." These selection criteria, constituting a "curable" patient profile, enhanced the program's potential for institutional and medical success, since the patients thus selected had a higher possibility of discharge and represented a lesser risk of "failure" that could be imputed to the program rather than to the patients' own etiological profiles.

Plymouth, located in an outlying suburban area, first impressed me with the sheer expanse of its grounds, which isolate from the surrounding highways and towns a spread-out collection of gloomy redbrick institutional buildings of 1920s and 1930s vintage. There were no security posts at Plymouth's entrances, and the grounds were not fenced off; the expanse itself sufficiently demarcated its spatial boundaries and guaranteed security. The patient wards inside the buildings were locked, however, and their windows were secured with grills; when patients had to be moved within a building for meals and activities, the doors to the building were also locked.[7] Houses stood at the periphery of the grounds, former residences for high-level administrators and professionals. The Latino day care center was in one of these houses, surrounded by foliage that emphasized its isolation from the rest of the institution.

The Hispanic ward, one of four in the building, consisted of a large activities area furnished with sofas, chairs, a television set, a record player, and assorted tables; a windowed gallery along the back wall gave this daytime space a light atmosphere. Additional smaller areas had been partitioned off with half-walls to separate a reading space with bookshelves and a smaller sitting room from the larger space in which patients could lounge, watch television, and listen to music. A door at one end of the activities area opened onto a corridor of offices, individual bedrooms, bathrooms, and a communal bedroom partitioned into several cubicles, each furnished with four beds; individual bedrooms had been assigned to women patients, while the communal bedroom was for male patients. This arrangement offset the reluctance of female patients to reside in a mixed ward and minimized sexual contact between male and female patients, a recurring situation in

closed institutions which staff in the Latino programs reported as highly problematic, however ubiquitous.

Staff would usually gather in the area in front of the doorway to the corridor to watch the patients when they were not engaged in any scheduled activity. I thought of this area as an informal panoptical spot, offering staff relatively unimpeded sight lines to all points of the activities area; the openness of the space also allowed staff the freedom to pounce whenever there was any disruption among the patients. This arrangement made both surveillance and control economical without the design feature of a formally constructed panoptical space. Such spaces need not necessarily be designed and physically inscribed, as Bentham (1995) emphasizes; they may be devised through individual movement and use of existing spaces.

Since I did not join the evaluation team until after the ward unification, I never saw the original gender-segregated wards; but descriptions I read indicate that all wards at Plymouth (predictably) had an identical layout. The two old wards, though, had been further gendered through their decor: the men's ward was painted beige and had illustrations of horses on its walls, while the women's ward tended toward pink and its art toward flowers. Fieldnote descriptions from the period also attest to the presence in these wards of a larger proportion of geriatric, highly institutionalized, and "regressive" patients than in the coed ward, to the extent that several of the research assistants expressed their doubts about the potential for success of the original wards or their effective ethnicization.

Ward bedrooms were off-limits to patients during the day, and programmed events and therapeutic interventions took place mostly in the activities area, where the furniture mimicked the layout of a generic living room. Patients would also gather to play table games in the gallery. During the daytime, the ward was populated by those patients who were not in the day program: the lower-functioning and more heavily medicated patients (the two tend to go hand in hand). Its program of activities was not regularly carried out; the most common official explanation for the lack of implementation was a shortage of staff to organize and supervise activities. But the low energy and short attention spans of these more dysfunctional, heavily medicated patients were also contributing factors.

The day program, in its homey setting, contrasted markedly with the institutional architecture and organization of the closed ward. As one of our research assistants once commented, it was startling to encounter such a cozy setting in a psychiatric institution—an assessment that I immediately shared when I first visited the day program. Patients who had been assigned to it were transported daily to a cottagelike two-story house whose comfortable furnishings and decor were frozen in the styles of the 1930s and 1940s, unin-

tentionally making it a perfect setting for Plymouth's elderly patients. Although I never asked the patients whether it had the same effect on them, the *casita* retained for me a Hollywoodesque aura, given its resemblance to the idealized domestic spaces constructed by the movie industry in the studio era.

My initial impression of a house that had been somehow abandoned and left untouched for decades was further enhanced by a detail in the organization of its internal space.[8] Two of its upstairs bedrooms had been converted into offices, but the third was duly appointed with a bed, chest of drawers, nightstands, and other domestic bedroom furniture; this bedroom and an adjoining bathroom were used to train patients in bed-making, grooming, and housekeeping chores as part of their Activities of Daily Living (ADL), a standardized scaled exercise widely used in practical rehabilitation for the disabled. Running the gamut from maintaining personal grooming habits to using public transportation and monitoring one's own medication schedule, ADL measure a patient's performative capacity in normal quotidian skills. Patients' degrees of ability to perform these activities are constituted as signs of emerging self-reliance and relative independence which indicate the alleviation and cure of mental illness. ADL were a common feature in all three of the programs as a documentable measure of patients' progress. But only Plymouth had the resources to simulate a domestic setting in which some of these skills could be "tested" to determine the adequacy of institutional plans for patients, including passes, home visits, and discharge.

The day program was unique to the Hispanic program, marking its singular status within the larger institution. Officially designed to provide continuity of care, the day program also publicly embodied social and institutional difference for the patients in the Hispanic program. It further de-homogenized institutional space and time for those who participated in it, even though they remained inmates in a psychiatric institution.

Since patients in the day program were ostensibly high-functioning potential candidates for discharge, the reduction of institutional signs and activities represented an attempt to constitute the program as a deinstitutionalized domain; it was nevertheless still configured as a therapeutic stage between actual institutionalization and prospective discharge. Staff assembled for their patients an ideal institutional life script in gradations and stages of progress, beginning with the institutionalization that signaled their serious mental illness, and leading to the ameliorative stage of the day program in which, at least for some time during their day, patients could be immersed in a simulation of the outside world. The ideal final outcome in this process was discharge, which publicly certified a patient's capacity for functioning outside the institution. The day program was the local reward for a

patient's progress in the transformation from illness to health, as well as its instrument and its measure.

Activities at the day program were different from those on the ward. The domestic organization of space—living room, dining room, den, bedroom, kitchen, a vegetable garden in the backyard—allowed for the assignment of patients to small groups in which they could participate more fully, get more individual attention from staff, and occupy themselves in activities that were different from those on the ward. Some of the activities were designed to capitalize on the home setting and to prepare patients for discharge: the schedule included cooking and English classes, the grooming activities involved in ADL skills instruction, and discharge groups in which placement plans were discussed. Patients were also expected to help with domestic tasks such as tidying up, gardening, and doing the dishes. I would find patients thus engaged when visiting the program; these chores were unselfconsciously performed by men and women alike, contrary to prevalent stereotypical representations about the traditionality of Latino gender roles.

In its third year as a demonstration project, the program instituted a third component, a discharge residence located in another house on Plymouth's grounds. It was initially designed to house three women patients, who would later be joined (after the evaluation had officially run its course) by two men. This component was soon plagued with administrative problems. Strictly speaking, these patients had officially been discharged and were not entitled to institutional care, so Plymouth could not assign funds for their support. The program managed, though, to capitalize on the support of upper-level administrators at the institution to alleviate these problems by redefining "discharge" so authority over these patients could be retained.

At another level, the establishment of this halfway house represented a further liminalization in a patient's institutional life script. The Plymouth program included a number of recidivist patients who would never be fully discharged because they had problems adjusting to the outside world; the halfway house thus accommodated those who could not totally achieve closure from their institutionalization.[9]

Plymouth had the most complex structure of the three Latino programs. The other two, at Northern Psychiatric Center and Jefferson Hospital, were mostly located in closed wards, and thus were more similar to each other than either of them was to the Plymouth program as a whole.

Northern Psychiatric: The Urban State Center

Northern Psychiatric Center is located in one of the five boroughs of New York City. It was chosen as the site for the second demonstration proj-

ect because it was a state facility in an urban area, and served a different kind of patient population than did Plymouth. Unlike the Plymouth program, the program at Northern was mandated. Latino staff at Plymouth felt that they had originated and consequently owned the program, particularly since they had done so outside the official institutional structure. Staff in the Northern program, in particular at its inception, attributed their problems of implementation to the fact that it was the product of official policy rather than of grassroots efforts.

Northern administrators claimed a very recent precedent for the Latino program at Northern: a Cross-Cultural Ward (CCW) established in 1986, scarcely a year before the Latino program was officially mandated; the initiation of the CCW in fact overlapped with the negotiations over the Latino programs. The CCW came about through the efforts of a non-Latina psychiatrist and medical anthropologist, and was purposely designed to treat immigrants who had problems adjusting to U.S. society because they were not fully acculturated. As a Latino administrator expressed it in an interview, the program had been devised to serve patients who suffered from *"desajustes culturales"* (cultural dysfunctions). This phrase codified one of those notions that prevailed among program staff: as a variation in their pathologization of cultural difference, intercultural contact was characterized as detrimental to mental health, a product of the deleterious effects that immigration and cultural difference presumably have on the self. Predictably, in order to sustain the establishment of the CCW, the institution capitalized on the argument that linguistic and cultural difference should be considered, ipso facto, barriers to effective psychiatric treatment.

The CCW itself grouped together patients and staff from a variety of ethnic backgrounds to provide "conditions of mutual understanding," as the institution's administrators expressed it—meaning language. This arrangement was not designed to develop culturally sensitive modalities of psychiatric care, as the Latino programs were. The only difference between the CCW and any regular ward at Northern was that staff and patients could communicate with one another in their native languages. There was no explicit conceptual dimension to its mandate; the CCW simply targeted the general goal of improving conditions of care for ethnic patients by matching them with caregivers who shared their language. Thus, while cultural difference was interpreted as a factor in mental illness, the arguments behind the CCW centered on linguistic difference as the relevant dimension for treatment.

With the establishment of the Latino program in 1987, the CCW's reason for being seems to have disappeared. Interestingly, though, it was never clear exactly how this happened. Staff assumed that, given the predominance of Latinos among its patient population, the Latino program was sim-

ply the CCW's successor. I never heard staff speak of experiences or knowledge culled from the CCW, perhaps because of its short life, although its existence enhanced Northern's chances for housing the new Latino program.

In reconstructing the history of the program at Northern, staff considered the CCW an institutional precedent that demonstrated administrative consciousness about the place of ethnicity in the delivery of mental health care; it was their closest equivalent to the actual grassroots Latino activism that characterized Plymouth's history. This perception was typically alleged by higher-level officials at the Latino program, however, not by lower-level staff. The CCW served to ground the Latino program in a constructed institutional history that burnished administrators' reputations; but the very same administrators capitalized on the fact that the Latino program had been officially mandated—that is, imposed—in order to reduce their own accountability for the lapses and shortcomings that impeded the program's development. Lower-level staff could less afford such views because they were the ones who felt the everyday effects of administrative neglect.

As in the other two programs, Northern's non-Latino staff resisted the establishment of the Latino program, and labor problems intertwined with ideological arguments about discrimination and preferential treatment. Since resistance there never took the institutionalized outlet of a union grievance procedure as at Plymouth, Northern's Latino staff attributed the problems to middle-level management's "obstinacy," which led to administrative boycotts in the assignment of resources. When newly recruited Latino staff were assigned to other wards rather than to the program, or an institution-wide recreational center went without material tailored to Latinos (both of which occurred during my fieldwork there), staff at the program characterized these incidents as racialized antagonism, thinly-veiled instances of official resistance to the program simply because it involved Latinos. Administrators I talked to, the alleged perpetrators of these injuries, claimed that they were constrained by institutional needs and budgetary problems. But Latino staff interpreted administrative actions within the context of national identity politics and ethno-racial hierarchies, which they believed were being reproduced within the institution—particularly as these actions were taking place in a city with a history of infamously complex ethno-racial politics. These interpretations were not exclusive to Northern staff, of course, but were shared by staff across the three programs. They were much more salient at Northern, however, particularly at the inception of the program, than they seemed at Plymouth, where interethnic conflict was reframed as labor struggles.

Though located in a city borough, Northern was as isolated as Plymouth from its environs. It adjoined a rather desolate area in a mixed residential and commercial neighborhood. But it remained an urban institution. Secu-

rity was much more evident: there was a guard post at the main entrance, and fenced grounds marked it off from its surroundings. Beyond lay mixed working- and middle-class neighborhoods whose presence was neither seen nor felt within the institution. Northern's atmosphere of totality and detachment from the outside world was emphasized by this proximity to noninstitutional life. Except for its recreation center, built in the 1970s, the institution was a conglomeration of boxy multistoried rectangles in the 1950s modernist style.

To reach the Hispanic ward, on an upper floor in one of these rectangular buildings, one had to traverse a long hallway, stopping first to ring a bell which would alert staff to open the heavy, solid door that led into its interior. (Because I had not been observant enough the first time I went there with one of our research assistants and had overlooked this bell, I spent several long minutes trying to make myself heard by banging on the door the first time I went by myself; it was only after meandering back down the hall that I realized my mistake.) Inside, the ward's physical configuration replicated the rectangular shape of the building: the space was organized into a central rectangle of offices with a glass-enclosed nurses' station at one end, surrounded by a corridor and then an outside rectangle of more offices, patients' bedrooms, bathrooms, a dayroom, a dining room, a visitors' room, and a seclusion room.

Within these nested rectangles, gradations of spatial access marked staff-patient distinctions. Patients were not allowed into the nurses' station without permission; this was the space used by paraprofessional staff for working, and by all staff for formal meetings, as well as for "hanging out." Permission was also required for patients to be in staff offices. But patients would frequently drift into these spaces to cajole, complain, or make requests from staff. Sometimes they were tolerated long enough to hold conversations with staff (including me: I once found myself addressing a patient's very acute questions about anthropology).

The dining room, bedrooms, and seclusion room were locked, and access to them was likewise regulated by staff. Only the dayroom and the corridor—which patients would pace continually—were spaces where patients could congregate and to which they had full access during the day. These were not totally unregulated spaces, however. The nurses' station, facing the dayroom, provided staff with a vantage point from which to maintain surveillance, and even though parts of the corridor were out of their line of sight, staff were quite attentive to patient movement. Since the offices of professional staff opened onto the corridor, they provided additional vantage points from which patients could be supervised.

The dayroom, a large open room, was furnished with sofas and easy chairs, most of which had been lined up against the walls or in neat, regu-

lar rows down the middle of the room—an arrangement that gave the space the forlorn atmosphere of a waiting room. A record player, television set, and a pool table provided unstructured patient recreation. The day-room was used for large-group therapeutic activities, but its most common use was as a sort of patient lounge for passive recreation and daytime sleeping, which only exacerbated its waiting room atmosphere. Other smaller rooms were used for small-group meetings and for medication and treatment.

The patient population at Northern was categorized as chronically ill, but not as institutionalized. Whereas Plymouth had no limit for its patients' length of stay, Northern had established an average time frame of six to nine months to "cure" its patients (or at least to discharge them). A good number of the patients on the ward had already been in the institution for several years, however, demonstrating the sheer formality of the administrative mandate. Others were "revolving door" patients who had been at the institution intermittently at different points in their lives. Staff offered a series of explanations for their lack of success in implementing the official time frame, all involving factors outside their control. Most commonly they alleged a dearth of adequate placement facilities, staff shortages that prevented the implementation of paperwork required for discharge, and the unavailability of relatives under whose care patients could be placed.

Raquel was the program's longest-secluded patient: a middle-aged Dominican woman who had been institutionalized since 1982 under court order. She had been acquitted, by reason of insanity, of killing her eleven-year-old niece, whom she had stabbed in the neck with a pair of scissors. Raquel was considered a high-functioning patient who generally tended to keep her distance from the rest of the patient population, claiming superior education, skills, and refinement of upbringing. Although she was deemed a good candidate for discharge, and she enjoyed outside passes and other privileges, she was not discharged during the evaluation period. The reasons advanced for Raquel's lengthy institutionalization included the legal complications of her case and an apparent lack of relatives to care for her in the United States. In spite of her usually high-functioning behavior, though, Raquel would "decompensate" whenever her discharge seemed imminent, indicating the degree to which she was dependent on institutionalization. The margin of doubt raised by these "regressions" legitimated the deferment of discharge. But the complexity of achieving it, in her case as in many others, undermined the effort to prove the medical and institutional worth of culturally sensitive care, at least as measured by the number of patients discharged. This problem affected all three Latino programs.

In terms of age, migration history, social conditions, and length of seclu-

sion, the patients at Northern offered a more diverse profile than those at Plymouth, and represented a less exact fit with the generic Latino "type" formulated in the efforts to establish the programs. Notably problematic at Northern, in definitional and institutional terms, was the presence of substance abusers, whom I learned to identify by the official designation of MICA (mentally ill chemically addicted) patients. MICA patients tended to be U.S.-born, younger-generation Latinos who were bilingual, English-dominant, or occasionally English monolingual in English. They were also notoriously hard to discharge, because of a Catch-22 situation limiting to the range of discharge options available: most drug treatment facilities exclude the mentally ill and most community mental health programs do not welcome substance abusers.

The presence of these patients was not officially sanctioned and was so highly problematic that it was often denied by program staff. Many of these young men and women were quite high functioning once "clean," that is, after withdrawal had weaned them from their addiction. They represented a problem of medical definition illustrating the ambiguities that attach to attempts to identify and classify "dysfunctional" behavior in psychiatric terms. MICAs raised questions about the etiology and manifestations of addiction vis-à-vis psychiatric conditions, as well as their assessment for diagnostic and treatment purposes. The exclusion of MICAs from both mental health and drug treatment programs underscored the problems of interpretation that accrue when institutions are faced with mixed categories that render ambiguous people's conditions and expected behaviors. These men and women did not fit the model of deviancy that either of these kinds of programs was designed to treat, but represented a compound sort of deviancy that staff viewed as particularly hard to control. MICAs acquired a powerful aura of danger and liminality in the imagination of Northern's staff, embodying a mixed array of stigmatizing signs.

The Northern Latino program, consisting as it did of a single closed inpatient ward, embodied a more traditional institutional model of totality. Although it had many implementation problems, and the politics of evaluation precluded our publicly comparing the programs, we privately deemed it the most "advanced" of the three in achieving its goals; we indicated as much in the final evaluation report, although we also carefully avoided rating any of the programs a complete "success."

In spite of the program's problematic beginnings, staff at Northern managed to overcome a series of institutional obstacles and engaged in a process of self-reflection in an attempt to articulate and produce certain "cultural" features that they then proceeded to integrate into their therapeutic approaches. Ironically, it was their achievement that led me to reconceptual-

ize the relationship between ethnicity and psychiatric care in more critical ways and triggered much of the analysis that occupies me here.

Jefferson Hospital: The City Program

During the negotiations to establish these programs, CHMH managed to extract a commitment from state officials to fund an inpatient program at an HHC facility, that is, in a city hospital. For CHMH, which concentrated its advocacy efforts in the city where many of its members practiced, it was politically important to engage the city agency in efforts to validate the concept of cultural sensitivity.

The establishment of a Latino program was first proposed to administrators of another city hospital; they turned it down, denying that the hospital served a critical mass of Latino patients. They also alleged that their staff were too sensitive to the implications of segregation in the concept of special services for particular ethnic populations, and were uneasy about the concept. Privately some CHMH leaders were less than charitable about this rejection; several characterized it as racist. According to them, the hospital did serve a large number of Hispanic patients. They also claimed personal knowledge of racist attitudes there. By the end of the evaluation period, though, the concept of culturally sensitive care had been sufficiently validated to lead several Latino professionals in this hospital to propose, fund, and establish a Hispanic outpatient clinic there, though not an inpatient program.

Administrators at Jefferson Hospital, a general city hospital in one of the city's boroughs, were then approached, and they accepted the offer. Jefferson's catchment area was predominantly Latino, though African Americans were a close second. Staff estimated the Latino patient population as 75 percent of the hospital's clientele, a figure that bolstered Jefferson's viability as a site for a Latino program. There was also a large proportion of Latinos among hospital staff, although the hierarchical structure of its psychiatric division was dominated by African American professionals at the time. Among the three programs, it was at Jefferson that the most explicit claims of racism and interethnic tension emerged. But it was also there that such charges were most often strategically deployed for the sake of validating entitlement within the institution's internal ethno-racial politics, which, in the actors' minds, replicated those of New York City.

Jefferson Hospital was located on a major commercial thoroughfare near two public housing projects, and housed in a red brick building that was barely twenty years old when the evaluation began. The hospital's physical appearance attested to the strain placed on its resources by its role as a pub-

lic general hospital in one of the city's poorest neighborhoods. People milled about in the common areas, lines for services were long, the building was physically deteriorating, and hygienic conditions were suspect. The hospital's straitened circumstances were obvious. I also heard stories, often quite mordant, which had achieved the status of urban folklore. One "joke" claimed that "everyone in the community knew" enough to try to be taken anywhere but Jefferson if they were mugged, or run over by a car, or taken sick. My personal favorite among these stories involved claims that muggers ran free through its floors accosting staff, patients, and visitors because security was so deficient.

Although I heard similar stories about other hospitals in the city, the ones about Jefferson were extreme, perhaps generated as a communal reaction both to actual conditions and to the institution's history—which was marked by political and financial scandals egregious even in New York City. But I also believe that these stories reflected a generalized tendency to rank public services lower than private ones. In a capitalist society, in which the use of money in exchange relations establishes the value of objects and services, what appears to be "free," and thus outside the "normal" relations of monetary exchange, is often suspect and subject to contempt.

Jefferson Hospital was not generally respected for the quality of its health care or the moral soundness of its administration. During our evaluation, it was plagued by rumors of corruption and medical inefficiency, which eventually surfaced and were subjected to official investigation; the institution constantly faced the possibility of losing its accreditation. Nevertheless, Jefferson was widely credited with pioneering unorthodox health care initiatives, notably the experimental use of *santería* and *espiritismo* in mental health care during the 1970s; it also operated a highly regarded acupuncture program for drug treatment in its immediate neighborhood.

While all three of the programs suffered from lack of resources and neglect in spite of declarations of bureaucratic commitment, these were a pervasive fact of life at Jefferson. Scarcity and disregard were very much a factor in the everyday operations and interactional dynamics in the Latino program, and were constantly mentioned by its staff. Limited institutional resources placed a premium on their allocation. Staff refracted the competition for scare resources through a discourse of interethnic conflict, an interpretation partially sustained by the ethno-racial composition of the organizational hierarchy in which the program was embedded, as well as by citywide politics of identity. Latinos at Jefferson tended to view the program as a reflection of the city's ethnoracial struggles writ small.

The general psychiatric facilities at Jefferson consisted of an emergency psychiatric unit, two closed inpatient wards, an outpatient clinic, and a mobile psychiatric crisis unit. When first proposed, the Latino program was de-

signed as an inpatient unit located in one of the closed wards; later on it was decided to establish a Latino outpatient clinic parallel to the existing general one. Documentation about the details surrounding the establishment and design of the program at Jefferson was sparse in comparison to the other two programs, but the rationale for adding an outpatient clinic seems to have been based simply on the number of Latinos already being served and the belief that they were being neglected by non-Latino staff at the regular outpatient clinic.

Unlike the other two programs, whose populations were relatively stable, Jefferson was designed to serve patients suffering from acute short-term mental conditions: people in full-blown psychiatric crisis. Official average length of stay in the ward was mandated at twenty-eight days, but as at Northern this time frame was mostly a formality. Jefferson staff also cited similar factors as preventing patient discharges, mostly involving the city-wide scarcity of alternatives. Moreover, precisely because of the crisis-oriented character of its services, it was more common at Jefferson for the program's patients to be homeless, destitute, and/or substance abusers. Patients were not transfers or referrals from other facilities, as was mostly the case at Plymouth and Northern, but people in acute distress picked up by the police, delivered to the hospital by frightened or exasperated relatives, or collected by Jefferson's own mobile psychiatric crisis intervention unit. The emergency nature of its patients' conditions allowed the inpatient wards little control over admission processes. At the Latino program, this translated into a reduced degree of latitude to enforce the program's ethnic and linguistic criteria of admission: if no beds were available on the other inpatient psychiatric ward for a patient admitted on an emergency basis, the Latino ward could not refuse admission, whoever the patient and whatever his or her identity or language competence. Staff at the program often jokingly compared their ward to the United Nations: Africans, Haitians, Chinese, Vietnamese, Pakistanis, and other members of the city's diverse ethnic communities could be lodged in the ward at any given moment.

My perceptions were that although this situation was certainly contrary to the Latino ward's stated goals, the program's purposes were in practice defeated by the kind of psychiatric treatment it gave its patients. Jefferson relied heavily on psychotropic medication. Of the patient population at all three programs, Jefferson's patients were the most visibly alienated in behavior, and their interactions with the outside world were largely curtailed, even if their alienation was temporary. These local circumstances of treatment were not conducive to facilitating, much less achieving, the program's goals, and as a result evaluators questioned the selection: perhaps Jefferson—or any other crisis-oriented institution—was not the most apposite site for developing a specialized ethnic program, given its mandate to treat

acute psychiatric conditions through universalizing biomedical means. We acknowledged the need for medication as standard psychiatric practice, and Jefferson's own local political need to assert a strong Latino presence; but of the three programs, it was certainly the least suited for essaying the complexities of implementing cultural sensitivity. Our assessments were generally quite strongly resented, provoking a difficult relationship between Jefferson staff and evaluators.

For example, I would consistently observe how patients at Jefferson were prone to spend their days sleeping in their bedrooms and to wear pajamas, which became a sort of institutional uniform for the program. Significantly, none of us ever saw patients in the other two programs dressed in anything but street clothes. When we documented this contrast in evaluation reports, program staff would often deny that the patients wore pajamas—only a very few did so occasionally, they would claim—and reports to the contrary were exaggerations made in bad faith, or the outcome of the "unscientific" method of ethnographic inquiry that we were applying. Alternatively, they would argue that if patients chose to wear pajamas, staff could do nothing about it because it was their right to wear whatever they wanted; staff were merely respecting patients' exercise of their rights.

I found these responses fascinating and, more important, culturally significant: they subsumed resistance to evaluative judgments by co-opting a jural discourse of rights and entitlements. The discourse of these Latino professionals was mediated by their need to achieve and retain interpretive control over their patients, the program, and the evaluation's outcome—especially since they resented our applying to their evaluation a nonpsychiatric interpretive frame grounded in a discipline not their own. The point about pajamas was not trivial, since the garment serves to mark publicly a patient's institutional status. It is one of several stigmatizing signs that is institutionally applied, while also providing staff with the visual means to identify patients and control their range of movement; pajamas are an attenuated alternative to the discredited method of keeping mental patients naked, as in the past.

Jefferson's outpatient clinic was directed to provide continuity of care for these short-term patients once staff on the inpatient ward determined that the abrupt, acute phase of their mental condition was over. The need for a Latino outpatient clinic was deemed particularly severe because there were no Latino staff in the regular outpatient clinic, even though it served a sizable Latino population.

Jefferson's two inpatient psychiatric wards took up the hospital's entire top floor. Located at opposite ends of the main hall, they were mirror images of each other. These wards were relatively isolated from the areas of general medical care, and were visited only by those who had business

there. The second ward had been designated the African American ward—and was referred to as such by program staff—but the Jefferson administrators never really implemented a full-fledged African American program as a counterpart to the bilingual, bicultural psychiatric program for Hispanics.[10]

The architectural layout of the ward was very similar to Northern's cookie-cutter institutional modern: a central rectangle surrounded by a corridor in turn surrounded by another rectangle where an activity room, bedrooms, bathrooms, and offices were situated. A nurses' station was similarly located at one end of the internal rectangle, with equally poor sight lines. Because its patients were so low functioning, a therapy aide was regularly posted at the opposite end from the nurses' station to survey the corridor. The ward's appearance was greatly enhanced by a glass-enclosed atrium located at its center, which was topped with a skylight that brightened the whole area; this atrium was used as a combination dayroom, activity space, and visiting room. Bedrooms were either single or double occupancy, and their doors were kept open because the programs' heavily medicated patients, were often in their rooms, though officially they were off-limits during the daytime. The bedrooms, the atrium, and the corridor comprised the regular patient spaces at Jefferson.

Reiterating its patients' medical distance from the inmates of the inpatient ward, the outpatient clinic was housed in the hospital's basement, a small, cramped, low-ceilinged warren of rooms that included a reception area, offices, and therapy rooms. One of these rooms had a one-way mirror into an adjoining therapy room for observational purposes, but neither of these rooms was ever used to my knowledge. Wall partitions were thin, and conversation easily penetrated them; everyone could hear much of what was said in therapy groups even from a distance. Whenever I visited the clinic, it was filled mostly with staff, but very few patients. Although the outpatient program reported a caseload of hundreds of patients, actual patient attendance and compliance with prescribed care were very low.

To add to its problems, the Latino program occupied an ambiguous position in Jefferson's administrative hierarchy. While the program's own hierarchy was centralized around a director's position, each of its components—inpatient ward and outpatient clinic—was part of the hospital's corresponding inpatient and outpatient divisions. These divisions in turn were defined as separate units for the purposes of both administrative and medical supervision. I once administered an exercise in the production of cognitive maps to different Jefferson administrators and professional staff in an assortment of positions both within and outside the Latino program. My request to depict their perceptions of the administrative structure in an organizational chart and flowcharts, especially lines of supervision and authority, produced a wide variety of interpretations of structural composition and staff position-

ing as well as of the program's relationship to the institution's other hierarchies. Most significant for me was how the director of the Latino program was variably positioned and, more often than not, excluded from lines of authority or subordinated to various non-Latino administrators.

This organizational confusion characterized the dynamics of the program: Jefferson's inpatient and outpatient psychiatric divisions were supervised by an African American and a Haitian professional, respectively, under the overall leadership of the acting director of Jefferson's psychiatry department, who was also African American. Both Latino and non-Latino personnel refracted this structural ambiguity through a lens of interethnic conflict that affected staff interpretations of the hospital's administration. Program staff's controlling perceptions revolved around these supervisors' perceived hostility to Latinos in general and to the program in particular. Problems in the implementation of the program were consistently attributed to African Americans' and Haitians' resistance to allowing Latinos "their due."

Program staff produced a more refined assessment of ethnic claims, reflecting their consciousness of the differences in the cultural location of the various ethric identities in question. But they could be quite exclusionistic in their struggle over what they perceived as finite material and symbolic resources. For example, Haitians were a strong presence among medical and administrative professionals at Jefferson. Latino staff maintained that Haitians were even more overtly hostile toward them and more resistant to the Hispanic program than African Americans; Haitians, staff would point out, "even claimed [the right to] a mental health program of their own." Once, when I commented to a Latina professional that Haitians certainly could claim as much cultural and linguistic otherness as Latinos in the United States, she responded, "It might very well be so, but there are no Haitians in Jefferson's catchment area. If they want to help their own people, why don't they go work in a hospital that serves a large Haitian population?" This statement aptly documents how political arguments for ethnic entitlement may be drawn from a variety of circumstances, not just "facts" of cultural otherness such as language, history, tradition, race, class, and so on. In this case, the argument was a variation on the numbers argument I discuss later. This Latina professional mapped ethnic entitlement as a product of the area's human topography and defined it in bureaucratic terms of the hospital's designated catchment area, "objective" criteria that legitimized Latino entitlement but defeated Haitian claims.

The program's first director, a Puerto Rican psychiatrist, strategically developed an administrative style that capitalized on the informal relations and personalistic networks of exchange within the hospital that had become a parallel structure to the formal administration. She was not the only offi-

cial to adopt that approach: the reliance on this alternative structure was widespread and quasi-normative at Jefferson. The program's second director, a Cuban psychiatrist, tried to adhere to formal channels. Unfortunately, neither was very successful in curing Jefferson's ills.[11]

The Issue of Ambience

It is evident from the preceding accounts that the three Latino programs were designed to embody a wide spectrum of institutional characteristics. They covered all the gradations of mental illness, from short-term, critical mental conditions to those that require long-term institutionalization. Their patient populations ranged from predominantly first-generation immigrants to the seemingly inevitable cultural mix that characterizes New York City. The programs were located in different urban and suburban settings and embedded within diverse administrative structures. Yet when staff at the three programs began to implement the mandate for a culturally sensitive ambience, they deployed markedly homogeneous signs and representations, their similarities limited perhaps only by local administrative responses and the availability of resources.

The proposals submitted for establishing the programs had already determined that physical features such as decor, food, and media were key components for inscribing a Latino ambience into the clinical spaces where the programs were sited. Staff duly complied in attempting to implement these and in providing "culturally appropriate" activities and services for patients, such as visits by Latino performers, outings to Latino events, and religious services in Spanish. A template of essentialized "Hispanicity" was already discernible in the act of foregrounding these particular dimensions of culture.

The use of Spanish as a common communicative and interactional code remained the major marker of identity for the programs, but the use of the other features contributed to providing a total institutional experience for the programs' patients. Components of ambience were used to ethnicize the institutional environment—perceived as "impersonal" and devoid of any cultural significance—and surround patients with symbols that staff were defining as core elements under the assumption that they were familiar and common to all Latinos. Thus subsumed under the rubric of a generalized "Hispanic culture," the elements that constituted a Latino ambience in the programs were material expressions of symbols of identity, deployed in the overarching strategy of contrastive definition.

For those who actually worked in the programs, these strategies were essential to the programs' development and legitimation for the interrelated reasons that I have introduced: they served to organize public and private

perceptions about the distinctiveness of the programs, to sensitize administrators in the sponsoring institutions to the value of inscribing cultural symbols in clinical settings, and to demonstrate the therapeutic effects a culturally sensitive ambience could have on psychiatric patients. Collaborators at the three Latino programs—their staff and patients, as well as outsiders—often expressed to us that their institutional life was "different" from that in regular psychiatric programs. This difference was consistently described as constituted by a certain affective tone that permeated the interactions and activities unfolding within the programs. Staff stressed that patients could make themselves understood better through the simple expedient of being able to use their native language. This improved understanding, staff maintained, reduced the usual inequality of staff-patient relationships.

For staff, the use of Spanish among themselves and with their patients conspicuously signaled the sharing of a common fund of cultural knowledge that facilitated the construction of interpersonal relations. The use of Latino music, the celebration of Latino holidays, and the provision of "native" foods similarly signaled the reproduction of ethnicity in a presumably decultured institutional setting. The infusion of ethnicity would provide patients with links to cultural experiences that had hitherto seemed threatened by the assimilating forces of the clinical setting and the dominant host society. It also signaled the staff's professional legitimation as enlightened mental health practitioners.

Many patients voiced similar assessments, but because of their radically different hierarchical positions, their reactions were more contingent, ambiguous, and negotiated. This difference was evident whenever we managed to pierce the staff's self-presentations and gain access to patients' reactions to the process of ethnicization. For example, when we administered the patient satisfaction questionnaire at all three programs, patients would use this power to try to negotiate privileges for themselves. Thus, one of the research assistants was instructed by a Northern patient to "change the answers" in his questionnaire. He was resentful because, in spite of his positive evaluation of the program, he had been denied a pass.

The implementation of the programs fulfilled different kinds of agendas for different participants. Latino professionals perceived the ethnic constructs and symbols deployed through the creation of a Latino ambience as the means to reconcile and achieve private and public ends. For patients, a Latino ambience could become the palpable expression of a cultural identity that had ostensibly been effaced, partially by the encounter with the host culture, and totally within the institutional setting. At the institutions in which the programs were situated, their ethnic ambience could mark them publicly as units entrusted with a special mandate. Finally, in terms of medical and institutional ideologies and practices, a culturally adequate ambi-

ence could potentially advance culturally sensitive assessment and treatment, and thus facilitate patients' discharges.

Signs and Representations

The most attainable first step toward creating an ethnically sensitive ambience, program staff determined, was to alter the institutional environment and create perceptual links to Latino culture through physical signs. The programs were liberally adorned with "Hispanic" motifs in the form of flags, portraits of historic figures, posters, photographs, and art from Latino countries. Articles and illustrations on current and historical events cut from magazines, newspapers, and books were posted on bulletin boards; particularly popular were stories discussing "what being Hispanic is about," media acknowledgments of a Latino cultural presence and its importance in the United States that could also be seen as prescriptions for performing ethnicity "adequately."

The relatively large numbers of Puerto Ricans among staff and patients often determined the nature of the decor. Indigenous motifs from Taíno culture proliferated; these motifs were regarded as "familiar"—and thus significant and soothing—cultural embodiments for all patients and staff. Many of the portraits pinned on the walls in the programs' wards were of Puerto Rican historical figures and artists. Patients at Plymouth, where the population was predominantly Puerto Rican, baptized their ward *"El coquí,"* after the minuscule indigenous tree frog whose call is pervasive among the night sounds of the island.

The director of Jefferson's program, a Puerto Rican psychiatrist, produced what I considered the most tangible representation of local attempts at intracultural domination. She commissioned a color photograph that was hung in the reception area of the outpatient program, depicting a large Puerto Rican flag and equally large national seal surrounded by flags from other Spanish American countries; because these other flags were on poles while the Puerto Rican flag was spread flat and centered, the others could hardly be seen. In this attempted portrait of pan-Hispanicity, the visually dominant symbols were thus the Puerto Rican flag and seal. Subordination produces such efforts to revalue publicly stigmatized cultural identities even at the expense of fellow subordinates (Fanon 1967).

These cultural motifs were conspicuously applied toward therapeutic ends, and their effects were closely monitored to ensure that they were fulfilling that purpose. At one of the programs, a community-based art education group held workshops to teach patients how to draw and paint indigenous motifs on cloth; the patients were also taught how to make native musical instruments from common materials, such as maracas fashioned

from Styrofoam cups. While ostensibly recreational, these activities were expected to exert a therapeutic effect according to the notion of milieu therapy. But the art workshops were short-lived. Staff initially explained that the institution had been slow to pay the group's fees. But the Latino administrator who supervised the program confirmed that the workshops had been terminated because they had been "too successful" at facilitating patients' self-expression. Patients had begun to paint "obscenities"—phrases such as "Fuck you"—a form of expression unacceptable to authorities, who saw such behavior as resistance to the socializing purposes of treatment, which could not be condoned. The need for subjugating and "normalizing" patients' behavior overrode any benefits that these workshops could provide, however "ethnic," therapeutic, or recreational their activities.

The three programs also strove to introduce "ethnic" themes in therapy groups, including discussions about Columbus's "discovery," the value of Latino identity as a point of commonality that brought patients and staff together, and expressions of ethnic pride and even militancy. Underpinning these themes was the effort to differentiate between Anglo and Hispanic cultures, and revalue the latter.

Native music—and dancing—was also used to help create a Latino ambience in both participatory and passive ways. Staff would play recorded Latino music for patients throughout the day, and in recreational therapy sessions patients were often urged to make music themselves. Improvised musical and singing groups made up of patients and staff were a recurring feature in the frequent celebrations of Latino holidays. These included holidays common to both Latino and U.S. culture, such as Christmas; others specific to Latinos, such as Three Kings' Day; and those exclusive to U.S. culture, such as Thanksgiving. The first and the last were generally celebrated in the programs, but paradoxically, holidays exclusive to Latino cultures were not much emphasized.

Determining whose holiday was being celebrated was actually a much more ambiguous task than staff had expected. Making choices and implementing them were affected by the tension between the overarching definition of Hispanicity applied in the programs and the need to accommodate ritualistic variety while remaining within the realm of authorized ritual activity. Thus, Thanksgiving is a holiday that is celebrated by Puerto Ricans (even on the island) but is personally foreign—except through media representations—and culturally insignificant to most other Latinos, especially among those who are recent immigrants. Particularizing the ritual was also an issue in the case of Halloween—All Hallow's Eve—which is of ancient European origin and was imported to the Americas, fostering a variety of locally produced, syncretistic celebrations with culturally distinct ritualistic specificities, such as the Mexican Día de los muertos. In practice, the festiv-

ities at the programs took whatever ritual form the dominant culture prescribed for them: pumpkins for Halloween and Santa Claus for Christmas.
Exclusively Latino holidays were not regularly celebrated in the programs,
with the occasional exception of Three Kings' Day, since doing so would
greatly have expanded the calendar of festivities.

Patients in two of the programs did participate prominently in the celebration of Hispanic Heritage Day, a holiday celebrated in many Latino
neighborhoods and communities, and when patients in one of the programs
participated in the local Puerto Rican Day parade, it served to forge links
with the local Latino community and enhanced the program's reputation
throughout the institution. The patients built a float for the parade, which
was later displayed on the institution's grounds. Allowing patients to participate in this parade, staff believed, would produce in them a sense of investment in institutional life which could be articulated in terms of ethnic
identity and pride. Indeed, when I visited the program shortly after this celebration, it was a favorite topic among the patients, who urged me to make
sure to look at the float. A similar sense of national pride emerged the following year, when the program held an official lunch to celebrate Hispanic
Heritage Day and the patients opened the ceremony—with the participation of local political figures—with a parade in which they marched into the
assembly room bearing the national flags of all the Latin American countries. Endearingly, the parade quickly lost its rigid martial orderliness
through the patients' palpable excitement.

Staff used foods associated with Latino cultures to enhance the specificity
of these cultural celebrations. Although institutional practice and economic
limitations precluded the serving of Latino foods on an everyday basis in
most of the programs, efforts were made to provide them on special occasions.[12] The symbolic dimensions of food, with its affective and cognitive
links to nurturance and subsistence and its universally recognized cultural
specificity, were thus capitalized on for the purpose of inserting ethnicity
into institutional practices. Celebrations created occasions when guests
from other departments of the institution were often invited to share in the
festivities. The programs were thus afforded the opportunity to reaffirm
their uniqueness within the immediate institutional community.

The use of media—Latino magazines, television, and newspapers—contributed to ethnicizing the institutional ambience but also to maintaining
patients' awareness of and links to contemporary conditions in the outside
world. Staff hoped in this way to counter the closed-off aspect of total institutions with access to a mediated outside "reality." They believed that the
sense of disjuncture from the outside world was exacerbated for Latino patients, since this world was presumed alien to them. Maintaining links to
their ethnic communities, however mediated, was designed to alleviate the

conditions of institutional life for Latino patients and enhance the possibility of therapeutic success.

In practice this goal proved hard to achieve. First, for economic reasons, the programs made do with reading material already available in the wards, and this material was mostly (if not entirely) in English. Over the course of the programs' implementation, budget cuts decreased the funding available for subscriptions to print media. Access to visual media such as videos and Spanish cable television was also affected. Staff would find themselves in the position of having to use their own personal resources—loans of equipment, home taping, renting at video outlets—to implement this aspect of the programs.

The deployment of personal resources was a common staff strategy for solving the problems caused by lack of special funding—problems that, higher-echelon administrators argued, were caused by the very uniqueness of the programs. When staff informally drew on their personal resources to supplement funding, it enhanced their sense of investment in the programs and contributed to the feeling of ethnic solidarity that the creation of a culturally sensitive ambience was meant to foster. It also replicated a we/they dichotomy common to interethnic relations, but in the institutional terms of Latino ("ethnic") program staff and patients versus mostly non-Latino ("nonethnic") administrators, who were perceived as unsympathetic to and unsupportive of the programs because of racism, discrimination, and the politics of identity that characterize the Latino struggle for public resources in New York City.

The incorporation of these features into institutional life thus contributed to the reproduction of ethnicity in a multiplicity of sites and relations. They were intended to produce an ambience of familiarity that would communalize daily life. In this sense, the creation of a Latino ambience represented an attempt to resist not only the acculturating effects of an institutional culture, but the assimilating force of the dominant U.S. culture as well. Language was central to this endeavor as the most overt defining marker of difference between Latino and Anglo culture. In addition, physical signs served to organize perceptions about spatial difference, and ethnically marked activities helped to differentiate the program from daily institutional experience.

Ambience in Institutional Life

The local native model of a monolithic Latino culture, deployed within all three programs in the specific material signs and symbolic practices that staff used, could not, however, accommodate pan-Latino diversity or even its expression as a U.S.-based experience. The model, variably implicit and

explicit, conjured a uniform patient population composed of Spanish-monolingual, traditionalist, conservative first-generation immigrants clustered under the overarching descriptor "Hispanic." The model was unmarked by the disruptions of local circumstances of history, class, race, age, origin, and so on that complicate the labels and orders of identity. The slippage characteristic of actual experience did not fit the abstract construct of homogeneous identity constituted as a political strategy of contrast.

For instance, many of the cultural elements employed in the creation of ambience were adopted from a highly idealized understanding of Puerto Rican culture. The prevalence of Puerto Rican cultural motifs reflected the predominance of Puerto Ricans in the New York City area and among the patient populations. But paraprofessionals—the people who interacted most on an everyday basis with patients—were also mostly Puerto Rican or "Nuyorican." These staff acted as "ethnic brokers" to translate the terms in which the program's mandate for cultural sensitivity was understood into those of everyday institutional life for patients.

The elements incorporated from Puerto Rican culture reflected its idealization as a traditional, unchanged society, sustaining the classic principle that ethnic symbols and the use of a native language forge perceptual links between an existing cultural community and an imagined historical counterpart (Fishman 1972). Certainly, staff at the programs were faced with a need for a standard to codify complex relationships and processes in the cultural representations they were importing into the programs. But their choices did not necessarily portray accurately or correlate with the Puerto Rican experience as cultural others in the United States, nor with other Latinos' experiences, even though staff were drawing from highly essentialized markers of identity that were communally recognizable. The construction of an ethnic identity at the programs, then, hinged on its representational functions of contrast with a dominant culture rather than on the actual sociocultural order within which the relations among all those involved in the programs were enacted.

Significantly, the model did not fit a younger generation of Latino patients—U.S.-born and/or raised—who represent what has been described as an interpenetrating bilingualism and biculturalism (see, e.g., Flores, Attinasi, and Pedraza 1981; Zentella 1990b). Such interpenetration arises from their experiences in the United States as members of culturally distinct groups that have been "othered" and have maintained, at the very least, a strong sense of distinctiveness from a "mainstream" Anglo/Euro-American culture that largely excludes them, yet at the same time reconstitutes them as "American ethnics" in a newly "multicultural" society. Because of the interpenetration of their dual cultural experience, by which they retain self-conscious links to a "native" culture outside the United States but also forge local ethno-racial identities within the United States, these patients could

relate to the ethnicized ambience in the programs and recognize its "American ethnic" distinctiveness. Their connection to the more traditional, essentialized features of the national culture model was more tenuous, however.

Staff itself were prone to such disconnections. For example, a bilingual nurse who identified herself as "Nuyorican" offered to resign when she was told that the program was bicultural as well as bilingual. Her logic: she was competent in Spanish and spoke it, but since she had been born and raised in New York City, she considered herself *bilingual* but not *bicultural*. During an interview, a program administrator who had likewise grown up in New York City pointed to a *cemí*—the stone image of a household god used among Caribbean Taíno Indians—and confessed that, although it had some aesthetic and cultural significance for him, it didn't carry the affective weight he *believed* it had for island-born Puerto Ricans. These perceptions were experience-based appraisals of identifiable markers of Latino culture, but they equally evoke the ongoing debate over the "content" and boundaries of cultures that have been constructed under conditions of immigration, colonialism, and subordination.

Because the model had been self-consciously formulated and deployed, it could and did function, to differing degrees, as an objectifying, unexamined, and homogenizing construct. It imbued staff with the feeling that "being Hispanic" was itself sufficient to render them culturally sensitive to issues of ethnicity in mental health care.[13] Further, Latino-ness was itself often predicated on having *native* knowledge of the Spanish language, a process that can be construed as the "naturalization" of culture. This conflation of linguistic competence and cultural knowledge effaced both linguistic and cultural diversity as well as the differentials of class, education, migration history, and other components of social location. These discursive contradictions underscore the commonsensical hold that ethnic culture and identity can have upon the imagination and attitudes of ethnic natives. But what I am suggesting is that these are also indications of how ethnicity can be strategically construed and capitalized on in a broader sociocultural context that both authorizes and rewards—within a dominant logic of subordination and the constraints it generates—the deployment of "culture" and "ethnic identity" for proving entitlement.

These paradoxes were not merely the product of political action. However intertwined these representations were with the need to legitimize the programs by marking ethnic identity through contrast, they also constitute what Woolard (1989:8) describes as the "publicly mediated meanings of group membership [that] inexorably affect the individual's daily experience of that identity." The context for their production, though, remained the therapeutic clinical setting, which shaped daily experience for staff and patients alike, as well as the institutional hierarchy of relationships and structured course of activities that organized everyday life in the programs.

[4]

The "Mother Tongue" and
the "Hispanic Character"

In order to validate further the ethnic constructs they had articulated, practitioners in the three Latino mental health programs devised an array of representational strategies. At the outset, though, they invoked two over-arching arguments to sustain their efforts on behalf of the programs. The first involved the demographic fact of an increasing Latino population in the United States. During the 1980s, when the programs were established, New York City's Latino communities had been replenished by an increased influx of immigrants from a variety of Latin American countries. This constituted Latinos as a particularly significant element in the city's political ecology. Advocates for the Latino programs drew from these demographics, exploiting what I call the numbers argument to sustain their establishment. In examining their use of this argument here, I mean to stress how public need and entitlement are quantified in the United States, specifically the mechanism by which demographic accounting is represented and translated directly into political weight by ethnic activists and others.

A second strategy drew from a body of psychiatric literature, most (if not all) of it generated by Latino researchers, including several who participated in the establishment and implementation of the Latino programs. This research dealt with the implications of using a native language in the course of therapeutic interventions.

Language obviously plays a primary role in psychiatric interactions for diagnostic and therapeutic purposes. In psychiatry, talk is a prime confessional technique for the abreaction of the self (Foucault 1978:67ff.). Staff in the Latino programs emphasized the importance of linguistic "expressive-

ness" as an interactional requirement for therapy. But since they were serving a population that displays a diversity of language competence, they needed to address how this linguistic diversity articulated with the centrality of language in therapeutic practices. In considering this issue, Latino program staff generated a notion that I began to think of as linguistic "regression." A body of research literature on bilingual behavior in therapeutic interactions was reframed and deployed in the programs to produce the locally dominant notion that while bilinguals may master two languages for purposes of everyday communication, they recur to their native language for "expressive" purposes. It became an article of faith among program staff that the "native" language for Latino bilinguals, *presumed to be Spanish*, became the most likely vehicle for the expression of psychopathology and thus a necessary component of diagnosis and treatment.

To some extent this idea ignored the fact that long-standing Latino speech communities are characterized by their multidialectal language repertoires. The array of linguistic competence among Latinos—who have accommodated to English monolingualism, especially in U.S.-born generations—challenges the assumption that Spanish is their "native" language. Ascertaining which language assumes the "native" function for therapeutic purposes was (and is) a complex proposition. Yet staff in the Latino programs posited linguistic "regression" not so much as a matter of a speaker's choice or preference (which would imply agency) but as the "naturalized" result of a universal process of language acquisition which constituted *a* primordial language as the retrievable nexus linking the adult self with its childhood and family experiences. Since childhood and family are themselves prime domains for the application of psychological and psychiatric techniques and interpretations, this notion constituted the "native" language as a highly essentialized component of the experiential matrix. By constituting Spanish as being more "expressive" than English—a characterization they also applied to the construction of a Latino "character"—Latino staff further bolstered the attribution of a "naturally" therapeutic quality to Spanish, and to Latino-ness, within local language and cultural ideologies.

The Numbers Argument

In his reflections on the rise of nationalism, Anderson (1991: 163ff.) characterizes the census as an institution of power imported and applied in nineteenth-century colonies to shape the ways in which colonial authorities imagined their possessions. Historically, colonial census categories increasingly became articulated in racial terms, that is, terms not of native provenance but generated by colonial officials in opposition to self-perceptions of

European "whiteness." Cultural identities were thus reified by the colonial power, processed through a classificatory grid that admits no ambiguity:

> One notices . . . the [colonial] census-makers' passion for completeness and unambiguity. Hence their intolerance of multiple, politically "transvestite," blurred, or changing identifications. Hence the weird subcategory, under each racial group, of "Others"—who, nonetheless, are absolutely not to be confused with *other* "Others." The fiction of the census is that everyone is in it, and that everyone has one—and only one—extremely clear place. No fractions. (Anderson 1991:165–66)

Colonial census takers thus engaged in a process of quantifying ethnic and racial identity to produce essentializing cultural maps of their domains. Current uses of the U.S. census are contemporary expressions of this colonial principle, by which identity, place, and entitlement are politically constructed and represented as a quantified basis for policy making, political strategies, resource allocation, and civic decisions. (I am arguing not so much for a spurious historical continuity as for an ideological one, rooted in a calculating rationality sustained by quantification.) Census categories thus index a wide variety of cultures and nationalities to constitute a classificatory grid by which the peoples so denominated may be defined, represented, positioned, and controlled by the state apparatus for a multiplicity of purposes. Not least among these purposes are policy making and resource distribution. But these representations can also be used by the people so denominated in order to penetrate and mobilize state systems of entitlement.

In the 1990 U.S. census the Latino population in New York City had increased 26.8 percent since 1980. While populations of Asian and Native American descent had increased in huge leaps and bounds over the same period—104.7 percent and 80.4 percent, respectively—their total number in the city was only 528,879, less than one-third the number of Latinos (1,783,511). By comparison, during the 1980s the number of white non-Latinos in New York City had diminished by 14.5 percent, while the black non-Latino population had increased by 9 percent.

The 1990 census also showed an increase in the percentage of Latinos in every one of New York City's boroughs, ranging from a high of 56.2 percent in Staten Island, generally perceived as the "whitest" borough in the city, to a low of 15.3 percent in Manhattan, where Latinos have been historically conspicuous, but have also been pushed out by gentrification and the erosion of manufacturing.[1] Population totals for black non-Latinos over the decade were generally lower than for Latinos. White non-Latinos decreased in all boroughs except Manhattan and Staten Island, where they increased by less than 1 percent. Total counts of the three major ethnic popu-

lations as New York City entered the 1990s was 3,163,125 for white non-Latinos, 1,847,049 for black non-Latinos, and 1,783,511 for Latinos; these three groups accounted for approximately 92.8 percent of the estimated citywide total population of 7,322,564.[2]

Mollenkopf (1993) notes certain contextual subtleties behind this quantification. He argues that the decrease among non-Latino whites in the 1980s did not indicate a diaspora of white New Yorkers fleeing a decaying inner city overrun by local "primitives," as the popular imagination has often had it. This assessment matches my own experiences in and of the city at the time. Unlike the 1970s, and even after the 1987 stock market crash that brought about economic recession in the early 1990s, the 1980s witnessed an influx into the city of people who profited from an expansionary economic period. But though the economic boom benefited some sectors, it exacerbated gaps in income and quality of life between the upper and middle classes (mostly white) and the racialized "minority" groups in the city, who tend to occupy the lower strata of the local class structure. These conditions placed a premium on political activism in the representation of vested interests, as well as for asserting collective claims on local public resources.

This is the demographic context in which Latino mental health professionals mobilized to advocate for the establishment of the psychiatric programs. More to the point, they explicitly incorporated and exploited demographic projections in the national census, which since the 1970s had anticipated the Latino influx that became so apparent in the 1990 count. Compounding other of their arguments, the numbers argument capped the rhetorical thrust of the Latino case. But it was only a part of that case; political ideologies prevalent in the nation played an even more prominent role.

As is widely recognized, public policy in the United States is entitlement-driven, and entitlements are organized in terms of difference. Difference, in turn, is established for the purpose of public policy through the quantification of groups of people who claim (or are imagined as sharing) a designated identity that qualifies their access to a specified portion of public resources. "Equal" access to resources and uniformity of means in the political and cultural imaginary of the United States are thus predicated on an assertion of difference in political processes, an apparent paradox targeted by critics of entitlement programs. Since the national apportionment of public funds is theoretically contingent on population counts, undercounting certain populations erodes the numerical base that justifies the "egalitarian" apportionment of these funds.

Redistribution in capitalist societies constitutes a paradoxical strategy for overcoming the inequities and vicissitudes of capital accumulation in an economic system driven by the presumably "objective" leveling effects of

[91]

the free market mechanism of exchange. As Nash (1989:23) points out, "The structure of redistribution gives vitality to the myths of equal opportunity, of mobility, and of justice" in modern states. Thereon rests the political weight that is attributed to quantification. Significantly, the 1990 census was challenged by various sectors of the population and became a politically contentious issue precisely because it had allegedly undercounted marginal populations such as "minorities" and the poor, thus eroding local claims to national resources.[3]

Beyond its validating force in redistributive processes, the numbers argument sustained other representations. Thus, the Latino programs were established in psychiatric facilities where a large proportion of existing staff and patients were Latino. "Need" meshed with local resources, and ultimately with entitlement, to facilitate favorable policy decisions. The national census sustained the argument that Latinos were the fastest growing among all other culturally distinct groups in the New York City area and its environs. This "objective" argument bolstered the "softer," "subjective" ideological and cultural arguments that the Latino professionals were deploying to persuade state and city officials to establish the programs.

In memoranda and speeches, conversations and discussions, Latino professionals cited the demographic trend represented by the census and its projections as "proving" both need and entitlement. The negotiations to establish the programs took place before the 1990 census, but the growth of the Latino population in New York City had already been identified as an inevitable trend. The 1980 census had shown a pattern of increase; the 1990 figures only confirmed the trend. The programs' appeal and propagandistic force among government officials were actually enhanced when the numbers argument was based on projections; it made a policy determination to authorize the programs appear foresighted, and thus particularly enlightened and timely.

This local numbers strategy was itself enhanced by contemporary perceptual changes in the national imaginary regarding the sociocultural profile of the nation and the strength of the different ethnic groups within its geopolitical spaces. Equally legitimated by the presumed objectivity of numbers, these perceptual changes were (and are) anchored in the belief that longstanding cultural and linguistic hierarchies are being revalued. Such is the case with the much-touted "Latinization" of the United States, which has presumably increased Latino cultural capital. In practice, such gains are illusory absent a corresponding class shift that increases the actual power of stigmatized speakers and ethnic social actors. Any apparent revaluation of subordinate status within dominant cultural and linguistic hierarchies is not a simple mechanistic product of sheer numbers, but is still subject to political and cultural contention (Bourdieu 1974, 1991; Gal 1988; Woolard 1989).[4]

[92]

The "Latinization" of the United States has by now acquired the aura of dogma. Darder and Torres dryly expressed the gist of this generalized perception, enhanced by the millenarian flourish so prevalent in the late 1990s: "Without question, the closing years of the twentieth century represent the culmination of major changes in the socioeconomic landscape of U.S. society. Nowhere is this more evident than in the 'Latinization' of the United States. Latinos currently number 24 million and, according to recent Census Bureau data, will become the largest ethnic minority group by the year 2009" (1998:3).

In its "positive" incarnations (beyond the force of sheer quantification), "Latinization" implies the recognition of Latinos as a major sociocultural group in the United States, the appropriation of Latino cultural elements as prominent components of the multicultural "mosaic" of national culture through their insertion into mainstream popular consciousness, and a *qualified* acceptance of Spanish as a medium of public communication. But this implication simplifies the historical complexities that characterize the Latino experience in the United States and the tenor of its long-standing relationship with mainstream Anglo-American culture. Vaunting Latino numerical strength and equating it with increased sociocultural power fosters the production of oppositional discourses as well as empowering ones—among others, those that support "English only" movements and legislation, the erosion of recognized language rights in key sociocultural domains such as voting and education, pervasive anti-immigration sentiments, and the persecution of undocumented alien workers on whom many regional economies depend.

Given these counterdiscursive manifestations emerging—or reemerging[5]—in response to an increased Latino presence that threatens dominant self-perceptions about the cultural composition of the polity, the "Latinization" phenomenon itself must be scrutinized, contextualized, and even challenged. Darder and Torres critique the facile assumptions the term "Latinization" codifies as it implies a degree of empowerment nonexistent in many Latino communities:

> Despite the increase in population and the political, educational, and economic advances of Latinos during the last 20 years, 30.3 percent (or 8.4 million) of Latinos continue to live in poverty. Latino workers continue to occupy the lowest rungs of the U.S. economy, finding themselves increasingly displaced and reconcentrated in conditions of structural underemployment and unemployment. (1998:3)

Ironically, even this challenge itself relies on the "objectivity" of numbers. My concern here is precisely with the continuous fetishization of numbers in the mobilization of ethnic political entitlement.

For Mexican Americans and Puerto Ricans, the pioneering Latino groups in the United States in terms of numbers, stability, and permanence, this belated discourse of "recognition" represented by allegations of "Latinization" has a sardonic ring. Yet this discourse of recognition has also brought us to a historic juncture for mobilizing and validating entitlement for all Latino communities in the United States. Contemporary multiculturalist discourses capitalize on the constitution of members of racialized groups as participants in the polity. As Nash (1989:23) argued about redistribution, this ideological strategy gives vitality to the democratic tolerance of difference that underpins principles of equal opportunity and participation. Latinos, in turn, necessarily feel compelled to exploit the semantics of power and identity embodied in these increasingly mainstream representations, however contestable (and contested) they may be. This mobilization is particularly crucial because the grid of identity in the United States has traditionally been articulated as a "black/white" dichotomy, in which Latinos and other ethno-racial identities occupy the ambiguous spaces between these poles (Blu 1979, 1980; Domínguez 1986).

Definitions of ethnicity must be localized for their analysis since they are contingent on historic sets of relations and long-standing structural conditions. But a degree of strategic essentializing, be it qualitatively or quantitatively derived, is often desirable or even necessary for the purpose of legitimating political action and mobilizing entitlement (Omi and Winant 1994:181, 188; Wilmsen 1996). The Latino mental health professionals involved with the New York programs were thus co-opting the grid of identity and entitlement embodied in the census for just such purposes. The numbers argument implicates a representational strategy in which Latinos are instantiated as a monolithic aggregation of sociocultural actors constituting a substantial part of the polity, a repositioning that should translate into considerable local political power under the dominant national ideologies.

Even though historical experience demonstrates that the effect of numbers cannot be taken for granted in actual political practice, it does not preclude their mobilization. In fact, experience encourages the mobilization of the numbers argument. And this capitalizing on the census also demonstrates its semiotic utility in a multiplicity of contexts; it gains value, through the exploitation of its polysemic character, beyond its deceptively utilitarian purposes as an instrument for demographic accounting. The apparent transparency of its purpose positions it as an "objective" measure that can be used to validate highly manipulable political agendas.

In further demonstration of the persuasive force of numbers in the public domain, the numbers argument from the census was buttressed by yet another kind of quantification. Latinos had been depicted as a population "at risk" for mental illness, implying that a larger proportion of Latinos than

other ethnic populations were in need of culturally and linguistically sensitive mental health services. Figures cited by Latino mental health professionals during the negotiations for the programs documented the rate of hospitalization for Latinos in psychiatric inpatient units at 34.5 percent, a proportion allegedly higher than the hospitalization rate for the white population (which goes unstated). Thus, over the larger numerical set of the census an additional quantifying grid was imposed to differentiate Latinos and constitute them politically and medically in order to enhance Latinos' entitlement to psychiatric programs of their own.

Language as "Regression"

Of all medical practices, psychiatry most relies on talk. As I have noted, speech is explicitly constituted as both a major psychiatric diagnostic device and an essential medium of treatment (Labov and Fanshel 1977:1; Ferrara 1994). For clinical practitioners who deal with patients who are linguistically "different," language is rendered problematic in therapeutic relationships, since the linguistic "mismatch" has the potential to affect both diagnostic assessment and the course of treatment.

From a sociolinguistic perspective, though, this notion becomes even more problematic when it defines language difference monolithically, exclusively in terms of standard national languages, admitting or contemplating no linguistic variation. Such was the case among staff in the Latino programs, where the notion of language mismatch rendered Spanish and English in dichotomous opposition, each configured as a uniform, monolithic standard code understood by and expected from all those who claimed one or the other as their "tongue." Language in the programs was being constituted solely, in Silverstein's (1987) terms, as exclusionary monoglot standards. Seldom explicitly considered were distinct forms of sociolinguistic practices, such as codes, dialects, registers, and diglossic usages, and other such patterns in linguistic repertoires that gain their meaning in the contextual and situational application of cultural and linguistic knowledge. Interestingly, staff in the Latino programs would note particulars of education and class among patients. But they treated variation in language practices as the product of idiosyncratic deviations from an *assumed* standard linguistic norm. These idiosyncratic deviations were deemed significant for their psychological import but not for their sociocultural and linguistic functions (see, e.g., Marcos 1988). Ironically, language was thus depleted of its sociocultural import in psychiatric programs that had been ostensibly designed precisely to reinsert sociocultural significance into therapeutic practices.

[95]

For me, the issue of mismatch became a particularly salient example of the clash between contending systems of belief—a "cultural" agenda of identity politics versus a "medical" agenda of "objective" scientific practice—which characterized the Latino programs. The concern with mismatch in the research literature gave rise to the notion of linguistic regression. It became important to me to examine how research on language was being construed by staff, since they explicitly based their local linguistic ideologies on it.

The notion of mismatch was not complexly problematized when Spanish-monolingual Latino patients and English-monolingual therapists interacted. In such cases it was evident that the linguistic difference would simply render diagnosis impossible and the therapeutic relationship inefficacious. Since most patients in the program were bilingual, such mono-lingual language conflict was of little concern. Even so, it is important to note that a recurrent concern for those of us on the evaluation team was how staff determined language competence. Estimates of the proportion of bilingual patients in the programs ranged from 20 to 60 percent at different points, and the actual number could have been even larger. Staff in the programs based their assessment of linguistic skills largely on an unsystematized combination of firsthand interactions with patients, self-reports, and speculation. Too often, competence went undetermined, and therefore unrecorded, or was based on commonly held notions that any ostensible indicator of Hispanicity—name, place of birth—accordingly entailed competence in Spanish. Patients born in the United States were generally categorized as bilingual, and those with other nations of origin were assumed to be Spanish-monolingual, whatever their actual code choice and ability.

Ironically, I always suspected that the determination of linguistic competence was rendered ambiguous precisely because of prevailing Latino linguistic practices shared by staff and patients alike. Staff's language assessments were complicated by the fact that many of them were themselves agile code-switchers, as is normative among members of stable Latino communities in the United States. Latino language repertoires blur, transcend, and challenge the monoglot character attributed to national languages (Flores and Yúdice 1990).[6] Code-switchers are often unconscious of the practice, and tend to underestimate its ubiquity in their own production.

Assessments of patients' language competence were also being generated under highly politicized conditions: staff would often assume greater Spanish competence than was the case in order to sustain the programs' Spanish-only mandate, as well as the stereotype of patients as tradition-bound monolinguals. As I discuss later on, reliance on psychotropic medication as

a treatment mainstay also tended to skew language assessments, since several of these medications can produce lethargy and slurred speech.

Conceptually and in practice, bilingualism confounded the issue of linguistic mismatch in therapeutic interactions. Staff at the Latino programs drew from contemporary research literature in which the "problem" of Latino bilingualism (and its ambiguous corollary of biculturalism) had been characterized as a source of "bias" detrimental to Latino patients.[7] This research recognized the evaluative functions that verbal interactions acquire in psychiatric practice. But these functions were still being assessed as important for their psychological (or idiosyncratic) rather than their sociocultural effects. In my view, the research drew from a deficient model of linguistic production, performance, and interaction.

The focus on bias generated two interrelated research issues. First, researchers hypothesized that linguistic mismatch increased the possibility of misdiagnosis. Second, the possibility of misdiagnosis made it imperative for researchers and therapists alike to attempt to assess in which of the two languages—Spanish or English—Latino bilingual patients would most accurately express symptoms (see Malgady, Rogler, and Costantino 1987).

From an anthropological perspective, a critical flaw that marred this research was the model of linguistic communication that it seemed to assume.[8] The researchers implicitly espoused a model of language production in which patient and therapist alike were reduced to alternating the roles of rote producer and passive receptor of a monolithic standard language devoid of any sociocultural function or agency. Intentionality was thus excised. The nature of linguistic communication as an interactive activity in which actual speakers strategically choose a multiplicity of linguistic forms within a particular sociocultural context in order to act upon the world went unacknowledged, perhaps even unrecognized. Language was reduced to narrow instrumental functions of expressing and perceiving psychological states.

The methodology used in this research was, for me, instructive. Carried out under the experimental conditions typical of scientific practices, it involved having Latino and non-Latino clinicians independently observe videotaped clinical interviews. Participants in these interviews were "matched" or "mismatched" according to ethnicity and language competence. The observing clinicians would then assess the degree of pathology "expressed" by the patients in each of the languages and compare their own clinical assessment to the one rendered by the clinician in the taped interview. The data generated were then subjected to statistical analysis. Research data, hypotheses, and conclusions were thus drawn from therapeutic interactions unlinked and disembedded from the actual sociolinguistic con-

texts and relations of production that shaped them, rather than from the ob-servation and documentation of naturally occurring interactions.

The subtextual implications underlying "mismatch" were somewhat transparent. Researchers quite explicitly presumed that English-speaking non-Latino therapists tended to misinterpret linguistic and cultural mani-festations and thus assess bilingual Latino patients as more severely ill than they actually were. This presumption suggested a solution to the first re-search issue—misdiagnosis on the basis of mismatch—through the obvious expediency of "matching" bilingual, bicultural patients with bilingual, bicul-tural therapists. This is what was to be implemented in the Latino programs.

Attempts to "solve" the second problem—judging how much pathology bilinguals expressed in either language—generated more complex and con-tradictory sets of hypotheses. These informed the notion of linguistic "re-gression" that Latino staff eventually articulated and applied in the pro-grams, however inconclusive or disparate the findings.

Researchers had initially concluded that bilingual Latinos "expressed" psychopathology more extensively in their native language (Del Castillo 1970). This conclusion was later contradicted, however, by research that seemed to indicate that English-speaking clinicians *inferred* greater psy-chopathology in bilingual Latino patients when they interviewed them in English than did Spanish-speaking clinicians when they interviewed them in Spanish (Marcos 1976; Marcos et al. 1973a, 1973b). This finding basically restored the issue of misdiagnosis intrinsic to mismatch. But to complicate matters further, using bilingual clinicians to evaluate interviews conducted in both Spanish and English, another body of research contradicted this second finding and reinstated the first: that bilingual Latinos express psy-chopathology more in their "native" language (Price and Cuellar 1981).

Rather than solving the problem, the body of research as a whole under-scored the complex interrelation of factors that affect the production of meaning and the exercise of agency (Hymes 1972). This research showed that the clinical researchers were focusing their inquiry on the *patient's* lan-guage as a typified locus of dysfunctionality that was taken for granted. Re-searchers overlooked the therapeutic intervention itself as a context-de-pendent speech event in which meaning is interactively created by two sociolinguistic actors.

Latino staff in the programs were aware of the many complex linguistic and cultural factors in play; this was evident to me in the field. But they nevertheless relied on the "mismatch" research and explicitly endorsed the hypothesis that bilingual patients express psychic symptoms more exten-sively and accurately in their native language. They also added an experien-tially based twist: that at moments of utmost psychic distress, Latinos recur

to their native language for its expressive value. This is why I ended up thinking about these issues in terms of linguistic "regression."

Latino staff in the programs represented this "regression" as common knowledge, often illustrating it with examples from incidents in emergency rooms and therapy sessions involving distressed or decompensating bilingual Latino patients. These patients were invariably represented as reverting to Spanish. For these Latino practitioners, this "natural" return to the childhood language, automatically presumed to be Spanish, indicated the psychic breakdown of the socially produced person. Linguistic habits were deemed "native" to the person, and were what "came naturally" in moments of psychic decline—as decompensation or in acute distress—representing the critical juncture when the psyche is divested of its socialization and returns to a "raw" state of psychic fragmentation as signaled by the onset of or relapse into mental illness. What had been socially acquired—competence in a language other than the native one—was thus construed as excised by psychic distress.

But the presumption that Spanish is the language of nature for Latinos is problematic. Bilingualism marks a speaker's ability to use two language varieties with distinct grammar systems, particularly when their use is essential in everyday social interaction and is integrated into the individual and collective speech repertoires available in a speech community. Whereas in some societies the habitual use of two languages or codes is kept separate, the authorized bilingual mode among members of Latino speech communities is the normative use of both English and Spanish within single speech events, and even within single utterances in the form of intrasentential code-switching (see Durán 1981; Amastae and Elias-Olivares 1982; Poplack 1981, 1982; Zentella 1981, 1982, 1990a, 1990b, 1997; Urciuoli 1996; Torres 1997).[9]

Determining the effect of psychopathology on an individual's linguistic repertoire and discourse, on the modes of talk that are authorized by the linguistic norms of the person's speech community, or on the degree of expression of psychopathology among persons with multiple linguistic competence and performance is a topic beyond the scope of this book. I do not dismiss lightly the concerns of the Latino professionals in the programs, who often expressed to me their interest in developing predictive instruments that would allow them to specify accurately the range of psychopathological content in patients' talk; such instruments would ostensibly allow them to assess the degree of symptomatology exhibited in either Spanish or English. The predictability of code-switching behavior (or of any other kind of linguistic behavior), however, has long been questioned, regardless of its regularity, appropriateness, and systematicity (Blom and Gumperz 1972; Gumperz 1982:82).

What concerned me was the excision of the dimensions of power that permeate the therapeutic relationship, particularly in situations informed by differential class positions, as was the case in the Latino programs. As a social activity, talk in medical settings plays a constitutive role beyond its expressive and communicative uses. The doctor-patient relationship reflects status and power differentials not only from the sociocultural perspective of economic class but also in terms of knowledge. I suggest here, as Cicourel has argued (1980), and as is amply recognized in the literature (Forrara 1994), that exchanges between doctors and patients should be conceptualized as speech events, given the interactive nature of language and its strategic use as a form of social action:

> The general point is to reveal the ways in which status and power are reflected in the specific language used for directing the interaction, talking about mental states, asserting something, clarifying a remark, requesting information, using imperative and declarative utterances, while also revealing the ambiguities of language that can lead to unclear inferences about the social meaning of an utterance. (Cicourel 1980:415)

Miscommunication and confusion—because of differences in social status, cultural background, language problems, and a lack of awareness of a patient's anxiety—affect the ongoing inferential process a doctor engages in during the exchange (Cicourel 1980:426). Medical knowledge by itself does not guarantee successful communication, and it is doubtful that the gaps that arise could be fully bridged through the simple expediency of "matching" therapists and patients by ethnic identity and language, especially when, as happened here, the actual bilingual practices among Latino speakers were being misconstrued.

The research findings, recognized sources of both disciplinary and practical knowledge among the Latino professionals in the programs, further authorized and legitimated the Spanish-only mandate. Language was thus applied toward political and institutional purposes, in the form of locally generated constructs about its therapeutic effects.

"The Mother Tongue" and Interethnic Hierarchies

An upper-level non-Latina administrator at Plymouth illustrated the importance of the Latino program there with a story about her experiences with a Chinese patient. In her account, the patient, who spoke only Mandarin, had a very poor prognosis and little chance for discharge because he was withdrawn and silenced within the monolingual, monocultural institu-

tional setting. But it so happened that this patient escaped from the facility and found his way to New York City's Chinatown, where he encountered speakers of Mandarin Chinese whom he enlisted in a search for his relatives. Although he never found any kin, he did locate people from his native village in China. Some months later, the Chinese patient returned to Plymouth to inform staff about the changes in his life: he was then happily living and working in the Chinese community. Most important, his mental condition had improved so dramatically that he did not need institutionalization or psychiatric treatment.

This narrative, with its quasi-mythical nuances of passage and transformation,[10] exemplifies notions I found prevalent in the Latino programs. This and similar narratives were used to articulate the relationships among language, culture, and mental health. The example of the Chinese patient is significant precisely because it was not about Latinos, thus underscoring how narratives about cultural and linguistic difference were articulated as universal signifying templates, constituting "objective" valuations about the relationship between otherness and mental health ideologies and practices.

The effect of the story lies in the correlation between otherness and mental pathology. Using one's native language and cohabiting with people who share one's cultural background are deemed essential to mental health and psychic integrity. A causal nexus is constructed linking estrangement from one's culture or language with psychic estrangement. Patienthood and institutionalization are represented as conditions that are structurally homologous to foreignness and migration: in this administrator's account, in order to act on his circumstances (i.e., to exercise agency), the Chinese patient needed not just to escape institutionalization—depicted as personally, culturally, and linguistically foreign to him—but also to go into the city, in a localized reverse migration. Once there, he had to reenter with travail the cultural enclave of Chinatown, where his culture and native language were being timelessly maintained and preserved, having been transported from their original locale and re-created as a symbolic (yet actual) space of sanctuary with curative effects. Cultural, linguistic, and psychic alienation were thus portrayed as experientially similar: the "cure," or transformation of the person from illness to health, for all three kinds of alienation then becomes contact with one's native culture and language:

> Language is important, but so is being surrounded by familiar settings. It is in times when we are most fragile, Ms. Holden [the non-Latina administrator] said, when we need a supportive environment, the need of "feeling comfortable with [our] own group." It is in times of weakness, as is the case of the [institution's] patients, when patients need most what occurred in their formative years and this includes familiar settings, language, memories, and other rele-

vant experiences. It is this that the [Latino program] attempts to offer [its] patients. Deep-seated beliefs cannot be removed totally from a patient's subconscious and these beliefs have an important bearing upon the patient's illness and future treatment.

Another core subtextual theme in the story, emanating from the correlation of otherness and pathology, is that kinship and family ties, relationships that are strained if not severed outright by institutionalization, are endowed with (and exert) a strong restorative effect that is universally recognized and desired. If these ties cannot be restored, culture and the native language can be constituted as their surrogate. This note of kinship and nurturing was reiterated in the metaphors Latino program staff articulated depicting language as a maternal, curative force. As a significant component of the array of childhood memories that individuals "carry" with them,[11] familial relationships—cultural, linguistic, and personal—are the historic ground from which psychic causality, and thus pathology, is to be inferred and constructed.

A basic premise in the production of these narratives was then that the familiar— behavior, persons, speech, norms—is key to the integration of the self lying at the purposive core of psychiatric care. This assumption overlooked the ambiguity and ambivalence of the familiar, which may be disruptive or alarming, as well as the fact that normativity and normality may be constructed, situational, and contingent. Highly complex domains of experience were thus simplified, their intrinsically paradoxical nature rendered soothingly consistent, their multiplicity simplified.

Staff at the Latino programs incorporated these premises into their own discourses about the therapeutic uses of ethnicity and language. Constructs of language were essential to the formulation of these discourses, as language remained the controlling indicator of difference (and thus of need) that distinguished Latinos from other ethnic groups. These assertions of entitlement were not exclusive to Latino staff, but were shared by others at the clinical settings. As much was exemplified in the narrative of the Chinese patient, advanced by a non-Latina as a validating narrative for culturally and linguistically specific services in general, and for the Latino program she supervised in particular.

Similarly, Dr. Smith, an upper-level African American administrator at Jefferson Hospital, specified language as the primary Latino identifier in order to distinguish between the Latino program and the African American one. In so doing, he indexed an identity array that differentially positioned local ethno-racial groups against a reified cultural standard of "Americanness."

As I described in the previous chapter, administrators at Jefferson had proposed the implementation of an African American program in their sec-

ond inpatient ward. But they faced a significant conundrum: What kind of "culturally sensitive" program could they develop for African American patients? As Dr. Smith argued, African Americans "were Americans" and "spoke English." His markers of difference and exclusion were thus somewhat vulnerable—the implicit assumption being that Latinos do not speak English and are not "Americans"—but his use of these boundaries was significant precisely for these assumptions. More important, Dr. Smith continued, issues of treatment concerning African American patients had "become mainstream" in the clinical literature. It was "not clear," he mused, what *cultural* issues, if any, might be relevant in treating African Americans. Although he admitted that it was "equally unclear" to him what cultural issues were relevant in the treatment of Latinos, Dr. Smith excepted language difference; the use of Spanish constituted a "clear" issue for him in the delivery of adequate mental health care for Latino patients. The lack of clarity in identifying relevant cultural issues for treating Latinos, he argued, was due to a dearth of expert research and practical clinical experience rather than the cultural assimilation that he maintained characterized African Americans—but not Latinos.

Dr. Smith's views were shared by Latino staff. Whether African American culture was "distinctive" enough to "merit" a specialized, culturally sensitive approach in mental health care,[12] the presumption that Latinos were invariably linguistically different guaranteed their distinctiveness. In his "native" ordering as an African American, Dr. Smith represented his own people as medical and institutional subjects who, from a "mainstream" perspective, were somewhat more familiar "others" than Latinos. For him, they shared a greater number of linguistic and cultural traits with other "Americans" because African Americans are "native-born." In fact, considering the diglossic situation that African American English represents in the United States (Dillard 1972), there is a strongly reductive monoglottic flavor to this administrator's assertion that "African Americans speak English."

The African American "place" in psychiatric ideologies and practices was defined by Dr. Smith in inclusionary terms: African American mental health care issues had been "mainstreamed," unlike those of Latinos. By this he implied that the African American sociocultural experience had been abstracted and systematized as psychiatric knowledge, embodied in standard modes of diagnosis and treatment, addressed through public policy, and resolved through the application of appropriate institutional practices. Regardless of whether such actually was (or is) the case, Dr. Smith and others believed that there was no need to develop culturally sensitive modalities of psychiatric care for African Americans—even though they recognized the political need to institute, however nominally, a specialized psychiatric program for them.

African Americans were thus positioned as cultural others who were, nevertheless, not such "other" others; they were construed as lying closer than Latinos to the unmarked "American" category. Latinos were placed farther away from the standard—although perhaps not to the same extent as the even more exotic Chinese escapee—mostly on the basis of language difference.

Latino staff similarly articulated cultural and linguistic difference by conflating and reducing New York City's ethno-racial diversity into a dichotomy that positioned Latinos at one pole (or even as an imaginary center), while non-Latino English-speaking whites, subsumed within the undifferentiated category of "*americanos*" or "*norteamericanos*," were lumped together with African Americans into an opposing pole of contrast:

> Lorenzo [a Puerto Rican caseworker at one of the programs] drew sharp distinctions between the cultural attitudes of Hispanics on the one hand, and "*americanos*" [white Americans] and Blacks, on the other. The latter two, said Lorenzo, do not share the same attitudes and values ("*valores*") as the Hispanics. As examples he pointed out that Hispanics are more "sensitive" ("*sensitivos*") toward children (i.e., they are not "hard" [*duros*] with them as are Blacks and Americans). Furthermore, Hispanics identify much more with the family than Blacks and Americans. The point is that Hispanic patients easily perceive cultural differences between themselves and non-Hispanic members.

On another occasion, Lorenzo expressed the relationship in slightly different terms: "We [Latinos] are like ham and cheese [in a sandwich]: Blacks on one side and whites on the other side. And if you look at it closely, the system provides a lot for this. In education, in hospital services, in services in general, there is a certain tendency for some to be favored more than others." Voicing resentment of a perceived hierarchy that subordinates Latinos and perpetuates their lack of access to public resources, Lorenzo applied a metaphor to codify a notion of difference that does not really distinguish between African Americans and white *americanos*. Both groups are assigned an identical term of metaphoric resemblance as the two slices of bread in a sandwich. The expression "*como el jamón del sandwich* (like the ham in a sandwich) is culturally significant, at least among Puerto Ricans. It describes the uncomfortable situation of being hemmed in, in a figurative space. The center is thus rendered ambiguous in Puerto Rican culture, rather than occupying the (unexaminedly) powerful position it is commonly assigned. The center, a contained yet besieged spatial imaginary, is not necessarily such a safe place.

These images of difference resonated with yet another overarching theme: emotional warmth and cohesiveness were deemed core traits in

Latino culture. This was a recurrent note among staff, often reiterated by Latino patients who would express a preference for the programs because, unlike in their previous institutional experiences, there were no *"morenos"* (blacks). These were allusions not to black Latinos but to local African Americans, whom they configured as non-Latinos, and often as merciless rivals in the struggle for material and symbolic resources.

An African American social worker who directed the program at Northern voiced very similar perceptions at different points in her year-long tenure:

> When discussing the [Latino] ward, Oprah stated that she didn't know what was special about the ward. However, she went on to say that they did play Latin music and [there] was more of a familiar atmosphere. She continued that during socials, everyone got up to dance and were more relaxed. I asked if she thought that this warm and familial environment was cultural and she said that she thought the staff "warm" *naturally*. They had elected to come on the ward and were therefore more likely to have a "help your own" attitude and be more committed to the patients. She continued that you can talk about your stereotypes, e.g., Hispanics are loud, like to feed people, like music, etc., but that on the ward you have a mix of loud and quiet people. The staff tend to get more emotionally involved with the patients and do things which go beyond their job descriptions.
>
> When she took on the job, [Oprah] was very much aware of the difficulties involved in her relations with the staff and the patients as a non-Hispanic. She has managed by being very open about her lack of [cultural and linguistic] understanding and soliciting help—translations, interpretations—from Hispanic staff. The very nature of the ward affects staffing, of course, because in trying to get nurses for short-term coverage in emergencies she gets reactions such as "Those people are going to be talking over my head," especially from African Americans. African American staff, she points out, are very different from Hispanics: they are "colder" in dealing with mental patients.

A Puerto Rican social worker at Jefferson similarly noted differences in patients' behavior, attributing it to the effect of ethnicity and language difference:

> In terms of patients, Hispanics tend to be more docile than Black Americans. Blacks tend to be more hostile, and Herminia conjectured that this could be due to their command of the language. I asked if English-dominant Hispanics are similar to the Spanish monolinguals. She said that many NY-raised Hispanics may be aggressive at first, but if you use good manners, they will feel ashamed of the way they acted. Black Americans usually won't back down. Respect is more a part of the Spanish culture.

These statements documented the construction of a localized ethnic categorical set which generally reflected New York City's politics of identity.

Non-Latino English-speaking whites were constituted as the dominant cultural group, while African Americans were cast as strong contenders for political and financial entitlement. The "we/they" dichotomy common to processes of identity construction in multicultural encounters was thus produced and reproduced among (and within) racialized groups engaged in ongoing attempts to position themselves productively in an adverse society. But since these representations of difference were being generated within a clinical setting, Latino staff embodied their perceptions about the cultural and political contexts of New York City in binary oppositions of affective attributes. The oppositional play revolved around "hard" and "soft" qualities of attitude and behavior: sensitivity as opposed to callousness, warmth against coldness, docility versus aggressiveness.

These attributions also influenced the ethnicization of the programs' ambience. Staff validated their choice of physical signs, representations, and activities by crediting them with the transformative power of turning the "cold" clinical environment into a "warm," familial space for their patients. They legitimated their choice in a discourse of emotions, but this emotional discourse was interspersed with a psychotherapeutic one. Patients with "flat affect" or who were "decompensating," staff claimed, could be "brought out" of their psychological state through ethnically marked singing, dancing, food, and celebrations, all of which shared an aura of gaiety, warmth, and commensality, as embodied in the Latino "character." The affective tone also ruptured the seriousness of purpose and formality of scientific, impersonal, "objective" clinical activities, infusing them with feeling. These were highly paradoxical undertakings: Latino staff were invested and oriented toward rational psychiatric care, but they were also subverting the clinical spaces by imbuing them with an affective tone defined as culturally specific to Latinos.

How language constitutes difference was equally articulated in metaphors of affect and nurture. Called upon to elucidate the place of language in psychiatric care, Latino staff generated constructs that went beyond the purely instrumental need for effective communication. In their constructs, effective communication itself was predicated not on knowing the systemic rules that organize language, but on staff's self-defined, intuitive expertise of the psycho- and ethnolinguistic functions that come into play when the native language is used *among natives.*

A controlling metaphor in these accounts feminized language as the primordial vehicle of emotional expression, reiterating the "natural" character of Spanish as *the* native language shared by all Latinos regardless of their actual code choice. Latino staff stressed the use of Spanish in psychiatric care because they attributed to it primordial psychological effects. After all, they would reiterate, Spanish constituted "the *mother* tongue." For them it

was the *innate* vehicle for emotional expression among Latino speakers and thus the most fitting instrument for the abreaction of the self required in psychiatry.

Several of the Latino professionals used a recurring metaphor that drew its force from motherhood to illustrate how Spanish impacts native speakers' perceptions and production. Words in Spanish, they proposed, carry different emotional connotations for a person of Hispanic extraction than the same words would in English. This was discursively presented as "common sense":

> [Dr. Calderón, a Puerto Rican psychiatrist] explained, as other staff members I've interviewed have also stated, that it is important to assess [patients'] condition[s] correctly, and provide better treatment [by communicating with them].
>
> But by "communication" Calderón was not only referring to what is [conveyed] through an elemental knowledge of grammar or syntax. It is important [she argued] to stress the importance of the "maternal language" (*idioma materno*) because it is *"el lenguaje de las emociones"* [the language of the emotions]. It is the maternal language which "better expresses" or conveys sentiments and emotions, which are important in a psychiatric setting. A patient who hears the word *"mamá"* immediately may feel a sense of emotional security; the term "mother" may not arouse this sense of security in the patient even if he/she were [able] to understand English. It may very well be that upon hearing "mother," *"no se [le] mueven las fibras emocionales"* ["a person's emotional chords are not shaken"].

One of Northern's psychologists produced a similar example, equally grounded in "commonsense" notions of childhood and maternal care:

> Violeta then provided an example of the importance of language, and specifically what she meant by language. Her example was that of a two-year-old who accompanies his mother to a shopping mall. There are a lot of people in the mall and the two-year-old and his mother are suddenly separated. Frightened, the toddler yells out, *"¡Mami!"* [Mommy!]. Though there very well may be many women in the mall who are mothers, and many who recognize the word "mami," only one will turn, recognize the voice, and head toward the toddler: his real mother. The mother will also recognize, in her son's voice, that he is frightened and will instantly allay his fears. And the toddler in turn will feel relieved as he is embraced by his mother, knowing that she will comfort him.
>
> In this example, Violeta [suggested] that, though important, the mere knowledge of the grammar of the language is insufficient for effective communication, that language is extremely important for it helps people to "communicate at different levels." These "different levels" relate to past experiences. The implication is that these are difficult to understand and convey by those who have not gone through these experiences, regardless of whether they

know the grammar of the language. Language, Violeta stated, is part of culture, but one can't "look at culture in itself"; knowledge and use of language has "priority" in the wards and elsewhere.

Motherhood, childhood, and the native language were thus constituted as a primordial affective matrix highly relevant in psychiatric settings for the purposes of therapeutic ministrations. Latino professionals posited that early memories in the form of life experiences, particularly significant in psychiatry, could be accessed only by those who share the language in which, presumably, they had originally been encoded. These emotional arousals were important for adequate treatment. Less acknowledged was the possibility that the native language and its uses have the potential to codify not just nurturance and care but also authority.

Professionals in the Latino programs thus reiterated the language argument used in the negotiations to substantiate the need for the programs. But they necessarily invoked another scenario. If curative effects reside in using a native language, it could be argued that any non-Latino who acquired competence in Spanish would be equally able to mine the psychosocial effects coded in the native language. But, though foregrounding language, the Latino professionals underscored the role of *native* cultural knowledge in therapy. Linguistic knowledge by itself was deemed insufficient to render psychotherapeutic communication productive. It was imperative that Spanish be enhanced with *native* Latino cultural knowledge. Latino professionals constituted "folk" versions of sociolinguistic principles which establish both language and culture as interacting mediating devices in the expression and interpretation of experience, and which recognize that communicative competence is contingent not on one's knowledge of language as system but on knowing how to deploy it in culturally effective ways (Hymes 1974).

Native cultural knowledge was thus constituted as an essential framework for linguistic competence—what a Latino psychiatrist described as a *"marco de referencia"* (frame of reference). This was indispensable for participants to understand clinical interventions *profoundly* and *accurately*, as required by recognized psychotherapeutic standards; by implication, to argue otherwise amounted to medical malpractice. A non-Latino Spanish speaker, Latino staff maintained, would fail to "understand" the nuances in the affective content of key native linguistic usages. This argument indicated an implicit acknowledgment that language ranges further than the immediate situational context and draws on shared background knowledge for significance and intelligibility. But it also reiterated how cultural and linguistic competence was being "naturalized":

Lorenzo began by responding, "How would an American that doesn't speak Spanish feel once he gets into the [Hispanic] ward? Would he remain mute (*'mudo'*)?" [He argued] that [i]t is absolutely important to be able to understand the patients, and in this case the American would feel frustrated in not being able to do so.

But even if the American clinician were to speak Spanish he would still not be able to communicate effectively with a Hispanic patient. Patients' attempt[s] at communicating with the clinician would be misunderstood (*"el intento de comunicación sería malinterpretado"*) since "customs" (*"costumbres"*) are very different. While this would be a problem in any context, it is especially problematic in the case of administering drugs (*"medicamentos"*) when patients would tend to agree with whatever the clinician says because the former would not understand the clinician. . . .

Spanish-speaking American clinicians do not really understand the culture of the patients in the [Hispanic] program and hence do not understand the patients (*"no entienden lo hispano /* they do not understand what is Hispanic"). Hence the clinician's interpretation of what is going on with a patient is bound to be wrong. Lorenzo made a distinction (one that has also appeared in other interviews) between being able to communicate by having knowledge of the Spanish language and not being able to communicate because one does not know the culture. . . .

Even if patients were to know a bit of English they would still not be able to communicate effectively with American clinicians. The English the patients, most of whom are poorly educated, would know would be "street English" (*"inglés de la calle"*) and this in itself would be a barrier to "communication." Patients, by speaking a little English, may be able to "communicate" with a clinician, but they would not be able to "reach" (*"llegar"*) the clinician. Implicit to the term "llegar" is to be able to *"identificarse con su clase"* [to identify with one's class].

These constructs about cultural knowledge were also shared by non-Latino professionals and administrators:

Why wouldn't non-Hispanic Spanish-speaking staff members function just as well in the [bilingual, bicultural psychiatric programs] as Hispanic staff members [might]? Ms. Holden [Northern's non-Hispanic administrator] was quite adamant in stating that the presence of [Hispanic staff] was of greater help to the patients. Mere knowledge of Spanish, she suggested, would not guarantee knowledge of the patients' culture and would therefore not allow for the same type of understanding. Many dimensions of meaning, such as those that are embedded in phrases or "sayings," may be lost as a staff member unconsciously translates from Spanish to English.

These commonsense notions acquired the character of shared cultural dogma, indicating that they were the product of converging local forces and

experiences. The value in these constructs lay in their seeming trans-parency, ordinariness, and shared nature; this was precisely what was being exploited. These constructs indexed how local actors were appropriating common stereotypes in order to revalue them for achieving institutional and political goals, rendering them intuitive validating arguments for the provision of culturally sensitive services. The lofty goal of cultural sensitiv-ity, however intensely political it might have been, was directed to empower both mental health practitioners and their patients.

But adherence to the principle did not mean that differential sociocultu-ral factors went unacknowledged. Latino heterogeneity was recognized, but significantly it was still subsumed under a common rubric of identity. This generalized identity is privileged; any factor that could suggest the ugly dis-ruptions of social conditions potentially emergent at the programs was ex-punged. Essentialist representations about Latino patients prevailed, as generated by a Latino administrator at Jefferson:

Returning to assessment and treatment, Chardón drew a distinction between medical personnel working in a laboratory and [those working] in a psychiatric setting. In the former, medical staff can pretty much control for all variables needed for their work, while in the latter they cannot. And one of the variables they cannot control but must deal with is language and culture insofar as [these influence] communication, and hence [the] treatment of patients. It is pretty much clear that adequate treatment can't be achieved if therapists can-not understand the patients. Yet culture is also important for communication, and in this sense non-Hispanic, Spanish-speaking staff members cannot be as effective as Hispanic, Spanish-speaking members.

Culture is important in any type of communication, Chardón suggested, but he preferred to stress the importance of culture in *non-verbal* communication. An example which he gave me concerned "typical" Hispanic attitudes toward authority and [their] impact on assessment and treatment. Hispanic patients, Chardón said, typically display an attitude of deference and awe toward those in authority. This is reflected in not staring directly into the eyes of the clini-cian (who is an authority figure) and of agreeing with whatever the clinician says or suggests. Now, these two attitudes may have an impact on assessment, diagnosis, and treatment recommendations. A patient [who] . . . does not look eye to eye and . . . lowers his head in front of a therapist unfamiliar with His-panic culture [may induce the therapist to] interpret this as a symptom of de-pression and of low self-esteem, which may lead to an incorrect diagnosis. The attitude of agreeing with the clinician (of not saying "no") may lead to incor-rect, or even harmful, medications [being] offered to the patient. The non-Hispanic staff member would not end up with sufficient information or input for an adequate treatment. A clinician who understands some of these atti-tudes will attempt a totally different approach (different questions and ways of

asking questions) from that of a non-Hispanic staff member. Chardón also cited the case of an Indian doctor who assessed a Hispanic patient and who, on the basis of linguistic terms, facial expressions, and ways in which the patient used his hands (Chardón could not remember the details) diagnosed the patient as hysterical and schizophrenic. A non-Hispanic staff member would also misunderstand patterns of family interaction. . . .

In addition . . . he stressed that not all Hispanics (he was really referring to Puerto Ricans) share the same culture. First-generation patients have attitudes and beliefs that differ significantly from second-generation patients, and he said that the latter share or form part of the "Puerto Rican culture in (i.e., of) New York."

Spanish language and culture were thus defined as a common bond among all Latinos and as that which can be expected to bind patients together. But though this sentiment was commonly shared by other Latino staff, their expectations were not just that these bonds could be applied toward the constitution of a community of Latino patients, but rather that they should render therapeutic benefits:

[Helena, a Puerto Rican psychologist] also said that one of the most important consequences of the use of [Spanish] within the ward was that it generated a sense of "community" among the patients, and that this helped very much in patient verbalization—an important aspect or dimension, it would appear, of patient therapy. According to Helena, patients who would otherwise feel uncomfortable in speaking and verbalizing their feelings have an easier time doing so in a Spanish-speaking environment; among Puerto Rican patients, many initial conversations begin with nostalgic thoughts about Puerto Rico and these, said Helena, serve as an avenue to express their present feelings, along with life events which occurred to them and which may have impacted upon their mental well-being.

Also, this sense of "community" . . . serves to generate social ties which seem to persist after the patients are discharged. These social ties and support networks which extend beyond the ward . . . are important . . . in that they ameliorate the social isolation which many experience after leaving the wards. The idea here is that this would perhaps not take place in a ward setting where English is the sole language spoken. These continued social ties and networks, Helena said, may also exist between patients and staff. She told me of a case of a discharged patient who went to live with some relatives in Manhattan. After some time, the patient, she later learned, regressed to his usual psychotic (and violent) state. His relatives, not wanting to call the police or another hospital, decided to call Helena to see what could be done about their relative. She in turn dispatched the Crisis Ambulatory Service to go pick him up and bring him to the ward.

A Latino psychiatrist and administrator at Northern further merged culture, language, and psychopathology into a medical model of treatment:

> Clinically, language is very important in psychiatric treatment: it is important for patients to feel comfortable in order to fully express themselves. A clinician who is not fully bilingual (and, by extension, bicultural)—someone who only knows a few words or phrases—cannot grasp *"la riqueza del lenguaje"* [the richness of the language] necessary in order to fully understand the background of the patients . . . and their [everyday] life experiences (*"la experiencia del diario vivir"*).
>
> But what about culture? Dr. Rueda believes . . . that we should constantly be aware of the fact that not all Hispanic patients share the same beliefs, attitudes, and norms. In addition, cultural beliefs regarding the etiology of what a clinician would believe to be mental illness or distress (he mentioned, for example, the belief in *"espíritus"* [spirits]) should be viewed as part of a complex of symptoms. That is, it is through symptoms that cultural beliefs are clearly manifested, or, to put it in a slightly different way, *cultural beliefs are components of symptoms*. Just as a physician looks at a variety of symptoms in order to diagnose a common cold or flu (runny nose and so forth), a psychiatrist interprets cultural beliefs as a part of a complex of symptoms which jointly point to a certain diagnosis. It makes very little difference, he suggested, whether certain cultural beliefs (or symptoms) are considered normal or acceptable: although this may be the case (i.e., that they are viewed as acceptable) this nevertheless would not mean that a patient is free of mental pathology. Mental pathology, he clearly stated, is "expressed by symptoms with a cultural basis" (*"expresado por síntomas con trasfondo cultural"*). Patients who arrive at [the institution] suffer from severe mental pathology, regardless of their cultural beliefs. What of the use of folk healers? Very problematic since, as he expressed earlier, not all patients would believe in the same "folk treatment" models. Although he did mention that he once worked in a very "liberal" hospital in Puerto Rico where *espiritistas* [spiritualist mediums] and psychiatrists would sometimes consult each other regarding assessment and treatment of patients.

In articulating the relationship between culture and psychopathology as he did ("cultural beliefs are components of symptoms"), this Latino psychiatrist constituted culture as a subject and domain of psychiatric practice. Cultural beliefs are paradoxically pathologized regardless of their cultural normativity. Cultural behavior is positioned outside the range of normality authorized by psychiatric practice and by the dominant culture. Also paradoxically, while pathologizing culture, he severed it from any connection to mental illness, which he universalized as a condition independent of any set of cultural beliefs: "Patients who arrive at [the institution] suffer from severe mental pathology, regardless of their cultural beliefs."

These inconsistencies illustrate the complexities involved in the task of conciliating culture with psychiatry. The task was particularly hard for mental health practitioners who had been socialized into the very ideologies and practices they were challenging.

Other corollaries emerged. Latino staff distinguished specific areas of concern about linguistic and cultural behavior related to the therapeutic setting. Staff working in the three programs offered a uniform list of practical and therapeutic consequences that could result from the lack of native cultural knowledge. These pronouncements acquired normative status among program staff and reiterated their concerns about miscommunication and misdiagnosis between Latino patients and non-Latino practitioners, as well as the effects of these slippages on treatment. These "normative" statements operated as exclusionary rules in the Latino programs. The boundary between "Latino" and "non-Latino" that was created on the strength of these local representations about both ethnicity and language was located in the affective dimensions of behavior, a cardinal psychiatric domain that could be accessed only through shared native knowledge.

Outside the boundaries thus erected stood both white Americans and African Americans, judged on the basis of their "attitudes" and "values." This representational strategy (*"we* are more sensitive toward children than they are because *they* are 'hard' with them," *"we* identify more with our families than *they* do") positioned the groups differentially. The overarching intrinsic attributes of the Latino "character" were positively located in personal warmth, caring, and consideration toward others. These depictions were often extended to unexpected domains. Dr. Calderón, the Latina psychiatrist who first directed Jefferson's program, was trying to get the Bronx Botanical Gardens to donate plants for the ward. When one of the evaluation research assistants asked her whether the African American ward would be getting plants too, she scoffed, indignant at the idea: African Americans do not "love," are not "addicted" to plants as Hispanics do and are. Of such minute typifying gestures was agency constructed at the programs.

Yet at another level, the constructs about ethnicity and language that these Latino professionals and paraprofessionals produced, revolving as they did around the revaluing of affect, underscored the paradoxical features of the emotional as a core identity component. Lutz (1990:69) points out:

As both an analytical and an everyday concept in the West, emotion, like the female, has typically been viewed as something natural rather than cultural, irrational rather than rational, chaotic rather than ordered, subjective rather than universal, physical rather than mental or intellectual, unintended and uncontrollable, and hence dangerous. This network of associations sets emotion

in disadvantaged contrast to more valued personal processes, particularly to cognition or rational thought, and the female in deficient relation to her male other. Another and competing theme in Western cultural renditions of emotion, however, contrasts emotion with cold alienation. Emotion, in this view, is life to its absence's death, is interpersonal connection or relationship to an emotional estrangement, is a glorified and free nature to a shackling civilization. This latter rendition of emotion echoes some of the fundamental ways the female has also been "redeemed," or alternatively and positively, construed.

The profile of Latino-ness produced in the programs could be equally construed as both imperfect and powerful because it was constructed around affective attributes and represented in feminized metaphors revolving around motherhood, nurturance, warmth, docility, respect, and meekness—a profile of individual and collective identity that is not necessarily prized in contemporary U.S. society. In a sense, these constructs were not very distant from everyday ones that play upon the patriarchal nature of the dominant host culture in which migrants are received and, as in the case at hand, served through public means.

But these constructs were directed precisely to exploit the power that the manipulation of affect achieves in therapeutic settings—which, after all, from a patient's lay perspective, deal primordially with the emotional lives of their subjects. Therefore, by stressing affect, these Latino professionals and paraprofessionals foregrounded ethnic difference to capitalize on ideological shifts in American policy making within a political context that prized discourses on cultural and linguistic difference. The discourses generated within the Latino programs could also be read as the construction of an ethnic character that redeemed its possessors because it opposed and challenged the attributes encountered in the cold, rationalized culture of the clinical spaces in which it was being constructed, as well as among the natives of the host culture. While constituting exclusionary representations, these discourses are not necessarily exclusive to Latinos, but are rather maximizations of ideations about ethnicity that are current in the multicultural ambience of the United States.

I do not mean to claim that these representations did not issue from experientially based assessments of what being Latino is about. Like the material signs deployed for the purpose of constructing an ethnic ambience in the programs, these representations were forged from an array of characterizing attributes that signaled the preferred terms of interaction within the ethnic in-group. The point is that, in the production of these representations, the mutual labeling and essentializing process that initiates the deployment of ethnic difference in situations of interethnic contact was used for overtly political purposes.

In practice, the everyday reality of the programs was more ambiguous, even while staff drew upon these representations to anchor the relationships that evolved among them, and between them and their patients. The practical development of the programs was also influenced by the constraints of operating within the times and spaces of public medical institutions. Ultimately, the construction of a stereotypical Latino patient as a psychiatric subject contributed to the reproduction of a medical ideology that systematized cultural traits and behaviors into an array of psychologized symptoms.

[5]

Occasions of Treatment

The strategies that Latino staff developed to produce "culturally sensitive" modalities of psychiatric care unfolded within the quotidian context of the programs. Life was organized into a weekly activities schedule similar to those in regular mental health treatment facilities; neither were they very different across the three Latino programs. Group activities punctuated patients' everyday lives to suffuse their institutional experience with therapeutic purpose. Activity schedules routinized a patient's day, providing an institutional framework for staff and patients alike. These activities embodied the totalizing technique of milieu therapy, as subscribed to by staff. They thus constituted a major field of action for the implementation of the programs' mandate for culturally sensitive care.

I focus here on the various group activities in the Latino programs, devised by staff in their self-conscious attempts to render patient experience culturally beneficial. This focus offers the best means of assessing the conciliation of medical and cultural agendas represented by the programs; it was in group activities that staff were most overt about their strategies for implementing their goals.

In order to apply therapeutic techniques that could be reconciled with their notions of Latino-ness, program staff soon concentrated on religious beliefs in *santería* and *espiritismo* as concrete cultural manifestations of and salient indices for the deconstruction of Latino psychic behavior. Staff perceived these religions as the Latino cultural traits most "exotic" to psychiatric practices and most inimical to the rational "normality" they wanted to restore among their patients. Since *espiritismo* and *santería* represented

the ultimate gap of meaning between Latinos and the dominant Anglo-American culture, these religions were also constituted as manifold, overdetermined embodiments of intractable difference that needed to be addressed through therapeutic applications.

There are, of course, concurrences and correlations between religion and psychiatry. As cultural systems of meaning, both construct behavioral causalities and aim for their remediation whenever behavior becomes inimical to personal or social purposes. Thus, both religion and psychiatry have devised rehabilitative practices for restoring personal and collective order, though these issue from such different ideological constructs about the world, human nature, and causality as to render religion and psychiatry seemingly extraneous to each other (Harwood 1977).

The deliberate focus on patients' adherence to *santería* and *espiritismo* as the etiological and interpretive frame for their illness was conveniently reinforced by its consonance with standards of psychiatric practice.[1] Contemporary treatment ideologies stress the importance of fostering patients' comprehension of the psychogenetic bases that have produced their mental condition, and define this as the controlling facilitating factor that renders treatment effective. Program staff thus felt that their concern for eliciting their Latino patients' self-perceptions about their application of psychiatric techniques was therapeutically appropriate. When patients produced responses defining and framing their condition in terms of *espiritismo* and *santería*, staff would explain to them how the psychiatric frame mapped onto the religious one, thus reconstituting psychiatry as a fitting replacement for religious beliefs as the more appropriate restorative source.

Ironically, in focusing on these religions, staff at the Latino programs were not being particularly innovative. These "folk" systems had already received a great deal of attention from the local medical establishment precisely because they constitute alternative frames of interpretation vis-à-vis scientific explanations of relations, events, and actions in the world.[2] This was, though, the first time that "folk" religions were being mined in inpatient programs, articulated with standard psychiatric practices, and systematized according to the mandate for cultural sensitivity, rather than treated as an adjunct therapeutic source. Staff attempts to achieve integration, however, confirmed my hypothesis that neither of these systems is amenable to an exhaustive translation into the other's terms, but rather both embody alternative symbolic modes for the constitution of meaning.

Although staff in the programs would sometimes treat religious beliefs as parallel resources for treating patients, more often they would "translate" manifestations of belief into psychiatric discourse, transmuting the bases of interpretation and understanding from the religious to the clinical. This is how they understood the mandate for cultural sensitivity. I

focus on instances of the use of *santería* and *espiritismo* in the Latino programs because these beliefs were particularly beguiling to the staff, who perceived them as concrete representations of an essentialized Latino culture even while they were also concurrently constructing them as antithetical to their own practical goals. Patients' cultural practices were thus refracted through a psychiatric lens that, paradoxically, contributed to medical primacy.

Yet another institutional mandate compounded the complexities of developing culturally sensitive care. A major institutional principle in the treatment of psychiatric patients in general is their eventual reintegration, their "mainstreaming," into personal and sociocultural "normality" as defined by society at large. This principle dictates the resocialization of patients to "prepare" them for reintegration into collective life. For patients in the Latino programs, this process explicitly required assimilation into the dominant mores of the United States. For staff in the Latino programs, whose purpose was the conservation and reproduction of ethnicity in a clinical setting, the mandate to "mainstream" their patients was obviously contradictory. Yet, ironically, Latino staff in the programs accepted, even defended, this mandate because it constituted the ultimate legitimation of the *curative* effects of their endeavors toward culturally sensitive care.

Underpinning the efforts of Latino staff to conciliate psychiatry and culture were definitions of standard behavior and ways of thinking that embody the cultural construction of typified symptoms of mental illnesses. As Fábrega (1996:11) notes:

> [A] society's knowledge structure pertaining to psychiatry incorporate[s] prevailing and traditional cultural standards and conventions about behavior; the illnesses described, their mode of diagnosis and technologies of treatment reflect conventions of how people should behave, how they (should or can) misbehave, what meanings are to be ascribed to behavioral alterations; and how such aberrations are to be shaped into normal channels of behavior, and how persons showing these aberrations are to be regarded and handled in the event "normal" behavior is reinstated.

As in regular programs, the actual assessment of mental illness in the Latino programs became an interpretive exercise of comparison fitting individual behavior to the psychiatric model. In conciliating ethnicity with psychiatry and implementing the mandate to mainstream their patients, program staff ultimately generated a mode of assessment that judged Latino behavior negatively by the cultural standards embodied in psychiatric models. Naming and defining are inherently exercises in power. Tech-

niques of subordinating power were being applied under the ironic guise of empowerment.

The programs' internal organization, institutional activities, and staff hierarchies provided the context for the process of identity construction that emerged. Because of their differential positioning within the local occupational hierarchies, individual staff were socialized into medical culture to differing degrees, with subsequent variations in their interpretation of the mandate.

Organizational Hierarchies

Mental health professionals and paraprofessionals are the recognized gatekeepers, interpreters, and rule makers of the mental health system (Estroff 1981:116). Publicly invested with an acknowledged store of specialized knowledge, they have the power to translate experience into the "technical frame of reference" of psychiatric ideology and practice (Goffman 1961:375; see also Foucault 1977, 1980). Within the bureaucratic structures that govern the mental health care system, this specialized knowledge ideally informs and legitimates policy decisions and actions.

The requirement for totally Latino staffing that had been negotiated for the programs was not defined merely as a practical need. As I have documented, underlying the requirement was the conviction that the conciliation of culture with medicine could be validly achieved only by "native" Latinos. The ethnic representations and the clinical elements involved in the production of the model had to be founded on the reinforced legitimacy of combined professional and native knowledge. These kinds of knowledge were configured as bolstering and legitimating each other, and were seen as ideally embodied in the cultural and institutional personae of the Latino professionals and paraprofessionals who would work in the programs. The application of this principle of native legitimation, as I discussed in the preceding chapter, was particularly salient in the local production of the language ideologies that program staff generated. At the core of the argument lies agency, the question of who is authorized to construct and perform ethnicity within a specialized institutional context that imposes its own validating criterion of "native" knowledge.

Even though Latino staffing was deemed essential to the medical, political, and cultural success of the programs, none ever managed to achieve it. It was better achieved at the level of professional staff than at the paraprofessional level. Administrators were markedly proactive in recruiting professionals, partly—but significantly—because professionals ostensibly pos-

sessed the kind of advanced knowledge required to produce culturally sensitive therapeutic models of care. The pace for recruiting Latino staff was thus shaped by occupational hierarchies, but also by epistemological ascriptions that differentially value particular forms of knowledge.

By professionals I mean staff members whose work functions required extensive educational training in a form of specialized knowledge within a particular valued subdomain of medicine and health care. Paraprofessionals were those who occupied adjunct positions vis-à-vis these professionals: they were assigned to discharge functions in the same occupational domains, but their work required less extensive training and specialized knowledge. Paraprofessional work was less valued precisely because of the symbolic capital attributed to extensive schooling and training, indexed by the achievement of advanced academic and professional degrees. Such tasks could be rather mundane, and many (if not all) were thought to require only relatively commonplace skills and knowledge; yet a paraprofessional position in the mental health field undeniably demands the ability to work in difficult settings and carry out particularly disagreeable tasks for an institutional population that can be exceedingly trying and hard to treat and "cure."

Professionals in the programs included psychiatrists, residents, medical doctors, interns, psychologists, psychology externs, and social workers. The paraprofessional class was mainly composed of recreation and activity therapists and their supervisors,[3] caseworkers, mental health therapy aides (MHTAs or TAs), and nurses.[4] Other personnel in the programs included clerical and housekeeping staff as well as occasional, mostly part-time staff such as ESL (English as a second language) teachers, MHTA trainees, and volunteers. Clerical and housekeeping staff were mostly Latinos, but occasional staff were not necessarily so. These staff were rather removed from regular patient contact, although in one program the Latino housekeeping staff were conspicuous for the close relationship they developed with the patients, which was acknowledged and appreciated.

Staff positions were not identical across the three programs, but they were similarly structured: they included a director[5] and, minimally, one psychiatrist, psychologist, social worker, and nurse, plus a number of MHTAs and activity therapists. The staffing was similar in Jefferson's outpatient clinic and in Plymouth's day program as well as in their inpatient wards.

Even though the Latino programs were demonstration projects for which special funding had supposedly been allocated, they were greatly affected by the recession of the early 1990s, which produced city- and statewide budgetary problems. The programs' budget situation was always somewhat ambiguous to me, enmeshed as the programs were with city and state politics, determined at a point in their history about which I had no personal

knowledge, and subjected to local strategies of capitalization. I did witness several situations in which program staff or administrators would strategically allege budget strictures when they failed to implement aspects of their mandate. Such was the case in the provision of Spanish-language media and the organization of Latino celebrations, which often suffered for lack of institutional funds, forcing staff to volunteer money, equipment, or food, or mobilize outside donors.

Staff vacancies were similarly attributed to budget problems. These funding issues supported staff claims that higher-level administrators discriminated against the programs either because they were racist or because they were not persuaded of the programs' worth. Withholding financial support fueled the tensions produced by local interethnic conflict and competition. Interestingly, though, administrators would sometimes mobilize the semantics of funding in other ways: they would assure staff (and evaluators) that the programs' special mandate would protect them from budget cuts and the city's and state's straitened financial situation; this helped counter recurrent rumors that the programs were about to be eliminated and precluded the flight of staff whose job stability would thus be threatened.[6]

In sum, staff shortages and turnovers in all three programs were common enough to sustain staff's everyday protests that their implementation of programmatic goals and the bureaucratic processing of patients' discharges were being disrupted. This, of course, curtailed their ability to "prove" the programs' "curative" worth. Staff at the programs also felt that it was valid to cite personnel shortages and budget problems as proof that administrators, and government officials were resisting Latino empowerment. To sum up, then, particularly among the Latino professionals at the top of the institutional hierarchies, New York's economic situation was consistently invoked to justify their inability to develop culturally sensitive modalities of care. At the same time, these accounts entered into the construction of a political discourse of differential treatment that could be mined to obtain personnel or resources from city and state officials.

Because paraprofessional staff performed the "dirty work" that institutional care entails their tasks brought them into intensive everyday contact with patients; professionals did not have such intensive patient contact. Paraprofessionals thus played an essential role in the ongoing surveillance and assessment of patients' institutional life. They also shared occupational, educational, and class affinities with the patients, who were largely from the urban poor and the working class, and these affinities reinforced whatever sense of ethnic commonality Latino patients and Latino staff might be expected to develop.

Patients articulated in personal terms their appreciation for those who cared for them on an everyday basis. It was common for patients to express

how the paraprofessional care they enjoyed diminished the role of professional staff in their treatment.

> Diana [a patient] spent considerable time praising *"estaffas"* [New York City Spanish for "staff"][7] It is clear that she sees them as the primary agents of patient improvement . . . : "Staff are like mothers to us. . . . [T]hey are the ones who orient us, who keep watch over us, who take care of our hygiene. . . . That book staff keep on each patient's life, of each patient's way of being, is what the doctors and the psychologists, the social workers take with them. Because they [professional staff] come to work [and] sit at their desks but they don't pay any attention to what the patient does. There are patients here who are picked up from the streets, who are sick, whom staff bathe, fix up, take care of. And you look at the patient after a couple of months and you have to exclaim, "And that was *that* patient!" . . . Then after patients are totally cleaned up, the social worker takes over to discharge them, because staff have prepared them and struggled over a patient so he can be discharged. . . ." She also gave an example . . . of how [the] social worker relies heavily on the advice of Vanessa and Norma [therapy aides] when considering [the discharge] of a patient. (translated from Spanish)

Certainly there were moments of tension between patients and paraprofessionals. But it was the latter who did the most to render the clinical environment familiar for patients and whose interactions with them imbued everyday life in the programs with its particular affective tone.

Goffman (1961) noted that lower-level staff in closed institutions act as a "buffer" between patients and professionals, insulating the latter from the hostile feelings and tense interactions that inmates exhibit with their immediate custodians, and draw patients' negative feelings upon their own heads. Although there was some variability among the three Latino programs, I discerned in them a clear-cut tendency toward inverting this process: paraprofessionals were generally more kindly regarded by patients than were professional staff. As I see it, this regard issued from a keen sensitivity to class, social location, and power hierarchies in Latino cultures, applied by these patients within the medical setting.[8]

Paraprofessionals constructed the mandate for cultural sensitivity in personal terms rather than in medical and institutional ones, mirroring the patients' personalization of their relationship.

> Sonia [housekeeping staff] asked me if I was coming to her birthday party. I asked her when was her birthday. It was December 15 and she was going to celebrate it in the ward. There was going to be *"lechón asado* / roast pig," *"arroz con gandules* / rice with pigeon peas" [and other typical Puerto Rican/ Latino food]. I asked her if this was going to be only for staff members. She replied, "Hey, what do you think? That I'm going to bring a roast pig here and

not give any to the patients? I wouldn't make them suffer. They love all that. And I want to celebrate my birthday with them."

Significantly, paraprofessionals uniformly maintained that the warmth of their interactions with the patients they cared for issued from their treating patients as "people" (as opposed to "patients"). They thus enacted the "warmth" that program advocates defined as an intrinsic component of Latino identity and aimed to medicalize by relocating it in the realm of human, rather than therapeutic, interactional strategies. For them, using cultural elements was a significant factor of mundane conviviality and human decency rather than a mandated instrument for making the programs culturally sensitive and therapeutically effective.

I am not arguing that paraprofessionals were "naturally" culturally sensitive as a function of class and culture, but rather that they were less socialized than professionals into viewing "culture" in essentialized terms, as a cluster of elements that could be "objectively" identified, extracted, and inserted into psychiatric principles and practices. Neither were paraprofessionals invested in this exercise as a conceptual calling and legitimating enterprise directed at enhancing political and institutional power. Paraprofessionals applied their own cultural knowledge in less self-conscious ways even while recognizing that they were participating in an important demonstration project and acknowledging its conceptual and practical nuances.

Constructing, Evaluating, and Treating Latino Patients

The programs' mental health practitioners, from a variety of disciplines, focused on documenting their patients' histories and institutional progress by mapping each one's life along an array of behavioral dimensions. All staff-patient interactions and interventions were inscribed and objectified in a series of specialized assessments. A patient's record was assembled from these assessments, constructing the patient's past and present personae both within the institution and in the outside world. A "team approach" guided patient treatment: each professional assessed the patient's history and actual condition to generate a joint treatment plan that organized the patient's institutional life and course of treatment.[9]

A patient's record embodied both synchronic and diachronic dimensions of being and experience: a patient's profile, rendered in and through a variety of disciplinary discourses, was produced by assessing her contemporary mental condition as constructed through her narrated past and projected on her future. These recorded life histories constituted an exercise in defini-

tion and interpretation: mundane incidents in a patient's life were deliberately elicited to gauge their effect as precipitating factors of mental illness. Life incidents were thereby redefined as psychogenic determinants.

Although staff at the programs believed that migration and cultural otherness were core psychogenic factors among Latino patients, an examination of patients' records showed that these circumstances too frequently went undocumented. Clinical assessments were couched in individualistic terms and constructed out of incidents pertaining to a patient's "private" life. Conjugal abandonment or conflict, complications in labor and childbirth, physical illnesses and conditions, the death of close relatives, parental neglect or abuse: these were the genres most consistently elicited and characterized as generators of illness. Assessment and treatment in the Latino programs were typified into individualized accounts that foregrounded the "private" dimensions of a patient's biography as the domain to be treated, following standard practice. In this sense, the professional assessments that were rendered at the programs showed no kind of overt "cultural" inflections, even under the local definitions of culture and understandings of where it should be located among the psychogenetic factors staff were applying.

The array of assessment categories used in the programs included psychiatric, psychological, social, medical/physical, activity, nursing, vocational, and nutritional evaluations. Generally these assessments were done when patients entered the institution and were updated throughout their institutional lives to provide the bases for medical decisions. Only the psychological assessment was not routinely done unless deemed necessary to rule out organic causes for a patient's mental condition, to "clarify" diagnoses in recidivist patients, or to evaluate patients under twenty-one years of age. I refer to this in particular as an indication of the highly medicalized nature of the treatment given Latino patients in the programs and staff's considerable reliance on psychotropic medication, which I address later on. While psychologists at the programs did lead therapy groups, the major mode of treatment in the programs predominantly hinged on medication.

Individual therapy was hardly ever available at the programs. I heard many Latino psychiatrists and psychologists in the programs opine that individual therapy was not indicated for Latino patients because they were not "reflexive" enough to make it work. This was a major reason why psychotropic medication and group therapy predominated in the programs. To me, this was a class-based justification, which also neatly sidestepped the need for more costly professional staffing and services. Ironically, these same professionals would claim that group therapy was problematic for Latino patients because "cultural" notions about privacy and morality precluded them from discussing intimate experiences and feelings publicly, thus further enforcing medication as the "chosen" treatment.

The assessments in each category were, of course, carried out by the professionals in whatever discipline was involved. These were then used to render a treatment plan to address a patient's "needs" and "goals." These needs and goals, both before and after discharge, were determined by each mental health professional on the basis of his or her own disciplinary constructs. Determining and analyzing "needs," "goals," "strengths," and "weaknesses" were further interpretive exercises in the application of disciplinary knowledge, and not necessarily wholly the product of a patient's self-reflection or volition.

Patients were not the sole source of information for these assessments. Whenever patients' relatives were available, program staff elicited information from them. In crisis situations, the police officers or paramedical staff who brought in the patient also became interpreters of the actual behavior that provoked the admission.[10] It was widespread practice, particularly in the case of patients with long institutional histories, to incorporate into their records information previously compiled by staff at other psychiatric facilities. Patients' histories were thus narrative composites of different people's perceptions. Rather than an expression about the self coming from a single source, no matter how multilayered and contingent any single human voice might be, patients' composites were multivocal and multitextual narrative constructions. Nevertheless, they were used to define the patient's *inner* reality, the psychic portrait of who the patient "really was," for the purpose of diagnosis and treatment.

A psychologist at one of the programs defined the treatment plan as "a multidisciplinary assessment that tells you what to do, when to do [it], and why do a treatment for a patient. It serves as a guideline to where you want to be headed with a patient." What to do was uniformly defined as totalizing modalities of treatment that articulated with milieu therapy:

> Verónica [social worker] told me that modalities [of treatment] were "interventions done to help the patient with his problem." In other words, interventions could be the specific types of therapies that occur. She defined therapy as "a goal-oriented interaction between a worker and a patient" [and] treatment as "encompass[ing] every interaction with the patient which helps him obtain a higher functioning level. Social interaction as takes place by saying hello to a patient and asking how his day was, arts and crafts in a group, etc., all can be considered treatment."

Over halfway through the evaluation fieldwork, we asked our research assistants to elicit from professionals in the programs their ranking of the different kinds of assessments in terms of each one's importance for their own practice. While some professionals selected their own, others crossed disci-

plinary lines to single out another. One of the psychologists, for example, responded that the social assessment (constructed by the social worker) was the most valuable because it gave the "developmental history" of a patient's childhood, the person's past and present history including "environmental" (patient's "social" characteristics such as occupation and education) and home situations: "It contains the *real* history of the patient" (my emphasis). This exercise showed, minimally, how conscious staff were of the complexities involved in the formation of the person and the construction of a particular life; it also underscored the problems involved in ranking one dimension of personhood over another, especially as represented in these assessments.

Whatever their discipline, though, it was for me significant that when professional staff were asked to rank treatment modalities, they agreed that psychopharmacology, the administration of medication, ideally complemented with psychotherapy, was the most important. This overwhelming preference was based on the therapeutic rationale that patients "had to be stabilized" through medication before any other kind of treatment could be effectively essayed. The dominant ideology in psychotherapy emphasizes the "self," a person's rational powers—however impeded and situationally inchoate—and individual autonomy as major enabling factors that lead to successful therapeutic interventions and mental health, making the reliance on medication, with its disabling physical and behavioral effects, highly paradoxical (cf. Estroff 1981:68ff.). As Harwood (1977:190) pointed out:

> Years ago Davis called attention to the clear correspondence between the values of Protestantism and the American mental hygiene movement. Among the assumptions that underpin both institutions he noted the importance of individualism, self-reliance, and rationalism. More recently Kiev, in contrasting psychiatric and other forms of psychotherapy, has underscored some of those same characteristics of the psychiatric therapies. He has noted "our own [Western psychiatric] emphasis on *the patient's* responsibility for his difficulty," the related belief in man's [*sic*] "destiny to master the environment," and "too much emphasis on cognitive changes and intellectual comprehension." (citations omitted)[11]

The use of chemical means to affect behavior is by now quite common in psychiatric practice. It fits with the contemporary trend toward biologizing mental conditions, which has driven the search for physiological causes in mental processes and in behavior. Kleinman (1988:73–74) has suggested that this biologization of behavior in psychotherapy is moved by economic interests and by a dominant system of cultural reproduction that stratifies disciplinary domains of interpretation and knowledge to position science and biology at the top of the epistemological hierarchy; biology, he argues,

is not intrinsic to the nature of mental illness itself. I could not agree more with him. It became for me a particularly paradoxical practice at the Latino programs, whose mandate and thrust were ostensibly toward acculturating mental pathology and changing modalities of diagnosis and treatment. In the programs' context, the reliance on medication seemed to nullify the avowed agenda. Kleinman's critique underscores the effect of a disciplinary stratification that likewise imbued treatment at the Latino programs with the medical culture in which the programs were embedded. The cultural "stuff" that was supposed to change standard practices was eventually subordinated to the alleged rationality of medicine and psychiatry.

Medication thus occupied the central place in staff's imagination and practices:

> [At a staff meeting,] another point of disagreement among the staff was medication dosage level. When Dr. Vélez and Dr. Marrero [residents] presented their cases, [other staff] would often shake their heads. Dr. Feliciano [psychiatrist] seemed a little incredulous at the low dosages being prescribed. [She] was most surprised at Dr. Vélez and said that considering he had worked in the emergency room, he should know better. Orlando [a caseworker] also commented that the dosage Dr. Vélez prescribed for a patient "*era para bebé* / was for babies"; he felt that patients had to be stabilized quickly in order for [discharge] placements to be obtained immediately. Dr. Vélez [defended himself] by stating that he had checked "with his attending psychiatrist" before prescribing the dosage. Dr. Feliciano told him that he could tell his attending [psychiatrist] that she had ordered the increase in dosage. Dr. Vélez also added, "*Yo me voy mañana y no quiero líos*/I'm leaving [the program] tomorrow and don't want any problems." Dr. Feliciano told Dr. Marrero that she had to remember that this was an acute short-term treatment facility and "we need to keep that in mind when prescribing dosages." If she prescribes a very low dosage in the beginning, and raises it incrementally, the patient could be institutionalized for two months before the accurate dosage is prescribed. The correct procedure, Dr. Feliciano continued, is to start the patient on a very high dose and then lower it.

Patients were socialized into preferring psychotropic medication, as shown in the following exchange during a psychiatric assessment session that was taped by one of our research assistants:

> *Psychiatrist*: What, what have you learned now that you've been here [in the program] from where you were before? . . . What have you learned here?
> *Patient*: What things have I learned?
> *Psychiatrist*: Aha (nodding).
> *Patient*: Nah, that there's help for those problems.
> *Psychiatrist*: Aha, isn't it so?

Patient: (nods).
Psychiatrist: And then, how can you solve those problems?
Patient: With medication.
Psychiatrist: OK. And by following treatment or not?
Patient: By following treatment.
Psychiatrist: This is why it's important for you to come to treatment once you're no longer in the hospital. [You want me] to discharge you because when you're discharged it's because you're stable. OK? And if you don't come for a follow-up, what's going to happen to you?
Patient: The same thing.
Psychiatrist: The same thing, right? You want the same thing to happen to you again or not?
Patient: NO!
Psychiatrist: OK. How do you feel now as opposed to how you felt at first?
Patient: Well. I feel well.
Psychiatrist: OK. It's a big change in your life.
Patient: Yeah.
Psychiatrist: OK. And your family has noticed this change in you?
Patient: Yes.
Psychiatrist: OK. (To evaluation team research assistant): That is, Raúl [the patient] is showing in this conversation we're having that he's conscious of his problem and seeks help for it. OK? And the solution he seeks is to stop those voices he hears and those weird feelings he has. He shows he's conscious of his problem when he says, "I know everything that's in my mind." There he's conscious that he has a . . . mental problem. OK? And that the only way to correct it is with . . . (Prompting patient)
Patient: Medication.
(translated from Spanish)

The technique socializes the patient to prefer a particular kind of treatment yet also to frame its course as engaging his own volition.

Medication groups, a common therapeutic activity in psychiatric programs, were an additional means of inducting patients into medication compliance and socializing them into the practice. In these groups, medical staff would instruct patients in the use, dosage, and effects of the psychotropic medications that had been prescribed for them; these sessions also allowed staff, in turn, to monitor medication effects and patient compliance. The Latina psychiatrist at Northern characterized the medication groups there as culturally sensitive because patients could be "open" and incorporate talk about topics she identified as patients' cultural beliefs:

"All this is possible because we do not have the barriers in this ward that other wards have for Hispanic patients. [In other wards] they wouldn't be able to talk about medication and their religious beliefs without feeling that they

would be laughed at or ridiculed. [We tell them] 'OK, this is your culture and your beliefs about healers but, on the other hand, there is this sickness called schizophrenia and this type of medication helps alleviate its symptoms. However, you can also use a healer to help process your treatment.' Accept their beliefs. They may not be able to change right away but it eventually sinks in."

[She added] that even she who is a Hispanic doctor often comes under fire from the patients for not being culturally sensitive. Patients have told her several times that she can't understand the culture because *"tú no sabes nada de brujería, lo único que tú sabes es de libros /* you know nothing about witchcraft, all you know comes from books."

Dr. Quintana also stated that she has noticed that patients are acting better after they have vented these feelings about witchcraft, etc. There was a patient who used to curse at staff. After going to a medication group and venting about *"el trabajo que tuve que hacer aquí porque esto estaba plaga'o /* the ritual cleansing I had to do here because the place was swarming [with spirits]," his behavior greatly improved and he doesn't curse at staff the way he used to although he still does curse at them.

Latino professionals at the programs constructed psychotropic medications as the rational counterpart of and adequate surrogate for the ameliorating effects that religious and ritual practices had on their patients. Patients were allowed to talk about such "cultural matters" as an exercise in a highly localized reproduction of ethnicity, for the (re)construction of their ethnic selves, or for reestablishing existential disjunctures. But they were primarily allowed to "talk culture" as part of their resocialization toward a therapeutic worldview in which the cultural was being constituted as an adjunct to the clinical. Patients resisted this, and their resistance was duly noted, but it was then reframed and articulated as a transient reaction that would be eradicated with further therapy, or defused through the therapeutic technique of talk, including talk that (as we just saw), constitutes medication as a salutary habit for patients to adopt if they really want to be cured.[12]

Activity groups also matched the mental health disciplines represented in the programs and were accordingly designed along disciplinary prescriptions. Thus the psychiatric assessment entailed medication groups devised to instruct patients on the use psychotropic drugs. Both the psychiatric and the psychological assessment (when done) entailed psychotherapy. The social assessment, the one most directly concerned with "environmental" factors, involved group and family therapy treatment. Activity assessments were compiled to monitor how patients behaved in recreational and occupational groups; their behavior was then clinically appraised to estimate their progress. All the structural components devised for patient assessment and treatment were thus organized around the specifics of each type of recognized disciplinary knowledge.

Non-medication therapies were generally delivered in group settings. The psychotherapeutic techniques that program staff applied in these groups drew on the therapeutic principle I have noted, by which the effectiveness of psychiatric treatment is thought to hinge on a patient's expressions of a subjected will, autonomy, sociability, and rationality. In most group activities patients were encouraged to voice opinions, discuss situations, and pass judgment on themselves and other patients, and were praised for actions that marked institutional adjustment and therefore curative progress:

> [At a group session:] Tomás [psychologist] then said that the TAs would give recognition to patients who are doing well and have been cooperating. Two TAs called out the names of those they felt had been good that week. Tomás asked those patients to join him in the center of the circle which they did hesitantly. When a small group of four patients had gathered, Tomás asked the TAs what they felt each patient should be complimented for. The TAs took turns explaining what each patient had done well: helping by setting up chairs for group activities, eating all their meals, waiting their turn to receive coffee and snacks, helping out with an older wheelchair-bound patient, showering without being asked, and being allowed to attend the day program because of their marked improvement. Each patient was applauded after their behavior was praised which caused much blushing and giggling [among them].
>
> The group took their seats and it seemed that recognition time was over when a TA asked a woman patient to stand. The two stood in the center and the TA gave the group a brief history on the woman. The patient didn't know how to hug when she was first admitted to the ward. She turned to the patient and asked her to give her a hug which the woman awkwardly did. At Tomás's suggestion, the group applauded this display of affection. The TA added that the woman was now more social, more affectionate, and had finally learned to hug. Again, a round of applause from the group.

Significantly, staff characterized participation in all of these groups as "voluntary." (A staff member once described them to me as "invitational.") Patients were not compelled to attend—in the sense that they were not forced or coerced. The emphasis on patients' agency issued from the dominant therapeutic principle placing the onus of treatment on the patient. Failure to participate, however, entailed negative staff assessments that were perpetuated in patients' records and reduced their discharge prospects.

This reminded me of practices in prison systems, where an inmate's participation in programs is interpreted as a sign of rehabilitation. Inmates in total institutions are generally perceived as desocialized, deviant actors who must be resocialized into normative behavior. Participation in group activities indicates sociability and an increased capacity to engage in social inter-

actions in sanctioned ways; it signifies as well one's subjection to collective rules and norms. Ironically, though, the practical reality in both penal and mental health facilities is that the monotony and regimentation of everyday life by themselves foster participation even when the activities being offered are not to inmates' liking and do not actually contribute to their resocialization. Inmates can also capitalize on this dominant belief in the meaning and value of participation, performing engagement strategically to gain institutional approval.

In any case, it was evident in the Latino programs that patienthood was being constructed in standard ways, as sanctioned by accepted psychiatric practices. The cultural was being reframed as adjunct to the clinical in the construction of patient personae, through the stress on medication as a prime treatment modality, and in the performative possibilities allowed to patients in therapeutic activities. But culture was also being construed as an intrinsic element of patienthood that must be tracked and, eventually, corrected for the patient to be considered "cured" and thus deserving of social reincorporation.

Fields of Action

Therapeutic activities included therapeutic community meetings, group therapy, "cultural awareness" or "cultural" groups, medication groups, recreational and vocational activities, reality-orientation groups, activities of daily living (ADL) sessions, family therapy and psychoeducation, discharge groups, and substance abuse groups. Except for the self-consciously "cultural" groups, they were all standard in psychiatric practice.

Actually, this array was more of the ideal type than otherwise. Though distinctively labeled, most therapeutic activities were formally and substantially alike: gatherings of groups of patients with staff, sometimes only paraprofessionals, at others just professionals; most times they were jointly led by both. Given the programs' strained financial situation, many therapeutic sessions were not held regularly even when officially scheduled.

Groups provided settings where the paradoxes that characterized the programs were enacted. At Northern, many of the Latina patients were predominantly middle-aged or elderly and mostly Spanish-dominant. They often converged in groups with a considerable cohort of younger U.S.-born or raised, English-dominant (or even monolingual) Latino patients, most of whom were mentally ill and chemically addicted (MICAs). These younger patients would often monopolize therapy sessions to talk about their lifestyle, their use of drugs, and their sexual experiences, to the discomfort of the older women.[13]

[T]he main topic throughout the meeting was a male patient's drug use and his ensuing [sexual] adventure during a weekend pass. Frankie [the patient] is a young male, apparently in his mid- to late 20s, and tall, with an athletic build. He has a history of drug abuse but didn't appear neurotic or psychotic. . . . Throughout the session, the main participants were Frankie, Manny [another young, English-dominant patient], Sandra [social worker], and Yolanda [TA]. The four remaining female patients and another male patient hardly had any input.

[T]he female patients were older and hardly spoke any English and most of the meeting [was] conducted in English—though once in a while Sandra interpreted. Frankie spoke very little Spanish so most of his story was in English. Therefore, [the other patients] felt excluded, confused, and were really not encouraged to participate by Sandra or the staff member. Also, the TA hardly spoke Spanish and the little she did know was mispronounced or grammatically incorrect.

The main topic was drug use. . . . One female patient walked out after about 25 minutes and commented, before leaving, that she had nothing to say.

Generational and linguistic clashes were not uncommon in group activities at the programs owing to the mix, among both patients and staff, of first-generation immigrants and "native" Latinos. Program administrators were required to submit data on staff's linguistic competence periodically for inclusion in the evaluation reports, but administrators applied somewhat monolithic categories of language competence: "bilingual," "English-monolingual," and "Spanish-monolingual." Multidialectal diversity as well as linguistic and dialectal dominance went unspecified and was mostly ascertained in practice.

These were likewise the language slots that staff applied to their patients. This categorization commonly gave rise to situations in which patients and staff who were allegedly bilingual actually demonstrated only a tenuous grasp of either Spanish or English. Whereas routine functional interactions could be negotiated in spite of the dissonance between recorded and actual linguistic competence, more crucial therapeutic interactions were problematic. In group situations, leaders usually handled the problem by using patients or other staff as translators; but translation, an unsatisfactory proposition in any case, affected the flow of communication and confounded nuances of significance. This outcome was particularly ironic since staff had so consistently articulated a language ideology that attributed intrinsic therapeutic force to Spanish.

Differences in linguistic competence would sometimes correlate with generational difference, as in the case of the group just documented, where age difference and linguistic difference were compounded, the communication flow was disrupted, and older patients felt alienated, diminishing the

group's therapeutic potential. Other times, the linguistic dissonance issued from dialectal diversity, which generated subtle gaps in understanding when, for example, speakers used their own national variety of Spanish, or a younger patient would use African American English.

As I have argued in previous chapters, most of the group activities in the programs were organized around talk and constitute speech events (Hymes 1972; Cicourel 1980). Their core purpose was the production of talk for therapeutic purposes, for the abreaction of the self so prized in mental health care. Patients were expected to "open" their selves through talk to staff and to the group at large as an intrinsically socializing and therapeutic instrument in group activities:

As I joined the group [therapy session], the focus was on a male patient who kept switching from Spanish to English and was saying that he wants to be cured, he wants to be patient, and he wants to be *"bueno y sano/*well and healthy," to be "normal." Dr. Ramos [psychiatrist] asked him what kind of patience was he talking about and how did it affect his life? The patient replied that he wants to be freed from something inside him that makes him go crazy and that's how he usually gets into trouble, he becomes violent. He wished to talk about who makes him crazy—another person inside him—but he didn't want to say his name because they would think that he's crazy. Pedro [activity therapist] told the patient that if he [didn't] feel comfortable saying what he wanted to say, he should not say it. Dr. Ramos interrupted and persuaded the patient to say whatever he wanted to say even if it makes him uncomfortable because "all of us here may be able to help you and we are for real, we're not phantoms." The patient, however, refused to say anything and didn't comment on Dr. Ramos's statement. . . .

[At a post-group staff meeting,] Brenda [psychiatric nurse who had participated in the group] told Dr. Ramos that she didn't agree with the way he had "pressured" the patient to disclose himself. Dr. Ramos replied that he felt it was necessary to get the information out to prevent further problems because "if we [don't] know what is bothering him, we [will] not be able to [devise] a treatment plan." Brenda argued that there was a better way to get the patient to open up and that is to do it in private. Dr. Ramos disagreed and said that the reason group therapy sessions are held is to have patients talk about their problems with other people so that they can get to trust others because one of the problems he finds with psychiatric patients is their inability to trust others, including significant others.

Zoraya [a volunteer and recovered psychiatric patient] agreed with Dr. Ramos and stressed the importance of "opening up" in the treatment process, especially when [one] is in the hospital where people are trying to help you and not harm you. Brenda still disagreed and said that people need their own privacy and shouldn't be forced to expose their feelings if they don't feel like it. Dr. Ramos said that we are looking for "group support": "One of the common

symptoms that patients express is fear. We should be teaching patients to form a trusting relationship with the group and not be scared of the group."

"Opening up," the abreaction technique of revelation that underpins psychotherapeutic practices, issues from the need to access what is inaccessible unless externalized through a variety of signs, material and symbolic, and particularly through language. But "opening up" implies making personal meanings public, and the production of signs is shaped by culturally defined boundaries between what is authorized as expressible in public as opposed to private domains. In this patient's logic, there were degrees of differentiation and revelation between unexpressed gradations of "craziness."[14] Staff articulated the situation exclusively in terms of psychiatric practices: the public and the private are here rendered not as cultural domains where production is controlled by the individual under different sets of rules and expectations, but as situations for which therapeutic practice has developed different techniques. The nurse's critique of Dr. Ramos's therapeutic approach hinges on its adequacy in the particular context of a group session: she expresses her preference for authorizing certain confessions during individual therapy and other kinds in group therapy. Issues about cultural definitions of the private versus public sphere or the normative adequacy of engaging in certain admissions are not addressed.

Therapy groups were thus occasions for patients to talk about what they faced inside or outside the institution in terms of their mental condition, feelings, and treatment. Staff defined and used therapy groups as collective activities in which patients were expected to display their skills of sociability and mutual help as appropriate indices of mental health:

A thin, black male patient was talking about his fear of loosing his apartment while being hospitalized. Yvonne [psychologist] appealed to the group for advice. [The patient] was advised by various patients to pay his rent, gas, and electricity. [A] patient suggested he tell his landlord that he was hospitalized. Another countered that he should not mention [that] he was in a mental institution because "people have very ignorant attitudes about mental illness." . . . This discussion took place entirely in Spanish. The first person to speak English was Carlos [activity therapist]. The patients followed suit: patients who had previously been talking Spanish switched to accented but fluid English.

An Anglo female patient . . . interrupted to inform Yvonne that she wanted to leave the group. Yvonne tried to dissuade her and the patient countered that she was not getting anything out of it because she didn't understand Spanish [sic]. Yvonne said that she would soon pause to translate and informed the group that the patient didn't know Spanish and periodic translations were needed. The group continued with the older patients generally speaking Span-

ish (though the bilinguals among them switched between Spanish and English) and the younger ones English. . . .

Silvio [activity therapist] tried to draw out a young English-dominant patient by asking her, in Spanish, why had she torn a painting from the wall and replaced it with her own painting. The patient shrugged her shoulders and remained silent. Silvio explained that the picture that the patient had torn down was somewhat mystical and occult. Another English-dominant young female asked the patient [in English] if the drawing reminded her of something that happened in the past. The patient answered, in English, that she didn't like the painting and found it ugly. Silvio asked who the patient shared a room with and a [middle-aged] patient who was sitting next to her raised her hand. He asked if the patient drew a lot and the older woman said yes, she drew well. Silvio commented that this patient seemed isolated and appealed to the group to make her feel more part of the ward.

Not talking or refusing to talk in groups—negating language—was interpreted as a manifestation of resistance. In clinical contexts, resistance is defined as pathological because it is interpreted as a patient's lack of insight into her condition as well as the refusal to engage in collective therapeutic actions directed toward curing it. Talking about her problems and publicly demonstrating consciousness about her mental condition documents a patient's self-awareness and mental health (cf. Mehan 1990). Staff at the Latino programs continually urged silent patients to talk and participate; otherwise, they believed, they could not fully assess the efficacy of treatment.

Groups were also designed to constitute staff and patients as a community, bound together in purpose and in action. This was most explicit in therapeutic community meetings, in which all staff and patients gathered to discuss institutional issues and events. These groups were devised as a forum for disseminating information, communicating program rules, announcing special activities, and introducing new staff and patients; staff and patients alike could raise everyday problems of interaction in therapeutic community meetings. These meetings thus helped to socialize patients into the more mundane dimensions of program life and the local normative requirements enforced for the maintenance of institutional order. They were also a venue used by staff to constitute clinical spaces, times, and persons as a cohesive institutional and ethnic aggregate and induct patients into the ethnicized, localized worldview that the Latino programs represented:

A lull of silence swept over the group which Tomás [psychologist] tried to break by asking how [the patients] felt living in a bilingual, bicultural ward. One woman patient said, "*Está bueno. Me dan de todo/* It's good. I get all sorts

of things," but the others remained silent. Tomás asked if they understood what he meant by a bilingual, bicultural ward and a woman said she didn't know what he was talking about. Tomás explained the term saying that they all share a similar culture, language, and past experiences, and that on this ward all are able to communicate with each other. The woman still didn't seem to understand and Tomás repeated the question to the group but no one responded. He dropped it. . . .

Tomás resumed the center and asked everyone to stand and join him. After some prodding, all patients and staff had gathered around him. He loudly proclaimed that they all needed to feel proud of being Hispanic and appreciate their culture. He then listed the various countries everyone is from and curiously mentioned Colombia first though no Colombians were present. He had them raise their hands in the air and yell, "*¡Somos Hispanos! /* We're Hispanic!" two or three times, after which a thundering round of applause followed.

The self-conscious insertion of ethnicity in group sessions was thus at times essayed as an exercise in explicit labeling to foster among the patients the construction of a Hispanic identity paralleling their own as inmates in a psychiatric institution. Other times, staff drew on cultural elements they assumed were "traditional" in Hispanic culture. This essentialistic approach was particularly used in "cultural" or "cultural awareness" groups, a genre that Northern developed explicitly for exploring ethnicity. These sessions were unique in that the agenda dictated that the clinical be largely contained and the institutional focus shift to the restoration of a collective memory rather than rest on individual pathology or institutional requirements:

Diana [social worker] said that they were going to talk about "*la Hispanidad /* Hispanicity." . . . Diana began by asking the patients if they knew who discovered America.

A Dominican patient raised his hand and began to tell the story [with a wealth of detail]: "*Todo empezó en la isla de Guamaní, que fue la primera tierra que pisó Colón. . . .* / It all began on the island of Guamaní which was the first land on which Columbus landed. . . ."

Diana asked the patients their opinion about the discovery of America taking into consideration their ethnic background. . . . She asked a Salvadoran patient what he thought about the topic. He answered, "*No recuerdo. Sólo sé que Colón descubrió El Salvador /* I don't remember. I only know that Columbus discovered El Salvador." Another patient said, "*Los españoles trajeron la caña /* The Spaniards brought sugar cane."

Diana said that it was a true fact that the Spaniards not only did bad things but also brought many good things: "*Los cambios traen cosas buenas y cosas malas. Malas porque causaron mucho daño y dolor, llevándose todo el oro y matando a muchos de los nativos de nuestras tierras. Buenas porque trajeron cosas como plantas y conocimientos de agricultura. Trajeron idiomas. ¿Qué id-*

ioma hablamos? / Change brings good and bad things. Bad because they [the Spanish] caused much harm and pain, taking all the gold and killing many of the natives in our lands. Good because they brought things such as plants and agriculture. They brought [us] languages. What language do we speak?" All the patients answered, "*Español*/Spanish." Diana asked, "*¿Qué religión tenemos la mayoría?* / What religion do most of us belong to?" Patients: "*Católicos*/ Catholic." She added, "*Entonces nos trajeron la religión y nuestras creencias. Por lo que todos estamos muy orgullosos de hablar español, de nuestra religión, de nuestras costumbres, y de comer arroz con habichuelas* / So they brought us religion and our beliefs. Thus we are all very proud to speak Spanish, of our religion, of our customs, and of eating rice and beans." A patient commented, "*El habla hispana es muy linda* / Hispanic speech is beautiful." Diana: "*Somos muy emotivos tambien*/We are very emotional also." . . .

A patient says, "*Es muy importante que la persona que viene a este país hable inglés porque se tiene que dar a entender con la gente de este país* / It's important for people who come to this country to learn English because they have to deal with the people here." The Dominican patient comments, "*Siempre nos la ponen difícil en este país por no saber inglés* / We're always given a hard time in this country because we don't know English." Diana: "*Los hispanos somos un grupo muy grande pero no hemos apreciado nuestros valores* / We Hispanic are a large group but we haven't appreciated our values."

Staff thus capitalized on constructs of historic bonds and cultural commonality to raise patients' consciousness about their ethnic identity. These efforts, often based on traditional cultural narratives or essentialist ethnic features, largely excluded patients' experience as ethnic migrants. In the session just described, it is the patients who voice more immediate concerns about their status as linguistic others—concerns that go largely unexplored. Sometimes, though, overt attempts were made to incorporate the immigrant experience into group discussions:

All the patients were now in the recreation room and the group was about to start. One patient . . . [asked] what are we talking about today? Wendy [social worker] told her that this was the cultural awareness group where they talk about Puerto Rico and compare it to life in the United States. Carmen [a patient] said that then they were going to talk about "*plátanos*/plantains." Everyone laughed. Wendy asked someone to bring up a topic. No one said anything until Carmen began to talk about "*verduras*/greens" and "*cuchifritos*/fritters."

Wendy decided to pick a topic. . . . She asked the group to talk about the role of the woman both in the U.S. and in Puerto Rico. One of the male patients began to say that women in P.R. wore "*batas*/robes," bring food and serve the men. Wendy then asked the patient if he was trying to say that there were differences in the women once they move to the U.S. The patient said yes. Carmen said that both men and women change once they move to the

U.S. She told everyone that when she was in PR, she and her husband were very happy. However, when they moved here, her husband took off with another woman, something that he would not have done in PR.

Gabriel [patient] seemed to disagree with what was being said. He claimed that there was no difference when women are in PR and when they're in the U.S. Miriam [patient] said that what makes couples change is the economic difference between here and PR. . . . When couples come here, the woman is forced to work to help her husband. . . . A male patient said that culture plays a big part in how women change when they come to the U.S. They want to be like American women and therefore, what they used to do in PR, they no longer do in the U.S. Another male patient said, "What do you want with a woman who sleeps all day, steals, and takes drugs?" . . .

Gabriel then began to describe his work on a farm in PR. . . . He was an immigrant worker [in the United States] and went from place to place to find work. However, he never changed nor did his wife. . . . Ricardo [said that] he came here at the age of 6 and is now 38. He visited NY and went back to PR to his grandmother [but] a big fight ensued between his parents and grandparents over his custody. . . . He was sent to NY with his mother who lived here. Now all his relatives have moved back to PR and he is here alone. . . .

Wendy then asked everyone if the houses in PR are as closed-in as the houses in the U.S. The patients got into a discussion on how everything was locked up here because if not they'd be stolen. . . . Ricardo said that in the U.S. there is too much murder. Carmen said that you find the same kind of thing happening in PR because it's been taken from the U.S. to PR.

Some of these sessions thus elicited experientially based accounts about ethnicity from the patients, who manage to engage in expert cultural analysis and critique. When patients are allowed to speak, their life accounts are complex, showing how situational, contested, and shifting the representation of ethnic experience can be.

Other times, ethnicity took on an instrumental, saliently political quality:

The [psychoeducational] group[15] was run entirely in Spanish and consisted of 13 women, mostly between 35 and 45. . . . All patients *seemed* to be Spanish-dominant or monolingual but this is difficult to gauge because many did not speak. Dr. Collazo's [psychiatrist] style in directing the group was to identify strongly with the patients as a fellow Hispanic. She would often say, "We Hispanics have a problem with———" and use herself as an example or talk [about] patients that she has.

One patient brought up [that] her children [speak] Spanish very poorly and she [doesn't speak] English very well. . . . Dr. Collazo commented that many Hispanic parents don't encourage the use of Spanish among their kids because "*venimos aquí y nos creemos que los americanos son lo mejor del mundo /* we come to this country and think that Americans are the hottest thing on earth. [Switching to English] We quickly lose our cultural and linguistic heritage and

all the beauty that it has." She emphasized the advantages of being bilingual [and] suggested that the mother learn English and the children Spanish by enrolling in language classes.

Dr. Collazo also discussed how she would like to see support groups formed among patients. She said that "in our countries" people are always helping each other; if you need a babysitter, your neighbor is always available and will not charge money. Many patients nodded and smiled in agreement. Here, Dr. Collazo continued, people become paranoid and suspicious of one another. She would like to see "the beautiful, help-giving aspects of our culture" displayed among group members. This is especially important for women, as usually the men work and have a network of friendships with co-workers outside the home. Women are more isolated but equally in need of friends. . . .

[Dr. Collazo went on] to say that she is both psychiatrist and director of the bilingual, bicultural psychiatric program and that her time attending patients takes her away from her administrative responsibilities. However, she is willing to do this because she is Hispanic and she will help out her people any way she can.

Dr. Collazo appealed often to the patients' sense of ethnic loyalty and cohesiveness to persuade them to attend the clinic. She emphasized that all of us are Hispanic, have a common culture and language, were raised similarly.

The discursive strategy used here is centered on a construction of otherness that capitalizes on the "we/they" dichotomy habitual in multicultural societies and in the expression of immigrant experiences. It is deployed at several levels: as a function of the program's special mandate, to elicit and share constructs of Hispanic ethnicity, for impression management, to establish common bonds that will enhance doctor-patient rapport, for ethnic empowerment, and in a mobilization of interest, to foster patient support for the program so as to guarantee its continuance. The native culture is imagined in personalistic terms. Exchange, for example, has allegedly not been monetized in Latino societies but is predicated on expectations of personal cooperation and reciprocity. In a neat inversion of the characterization of Latino culture as a psychogenic factor, life in the United States is rendered as psychogenic because its materialism, self-centered individualism, and impersonality vitiate basic decent humanity. Rather than its being Hispanic culture and character that are the site of production of "stress indicators," it is the host culture that is represented as the causative factor in the production of mental illness ("here people become paranoid and suspicious of each other"). The subject self-positioning of Hispanics as inferior others is critiqued ("we come to this country and think that Americans are the hottest thing on earth") in an attempt to revalue Hispanicity and dismantle the hierarchical relations between the two cultures.

Chapter 5

Permutations of Experience

In group activities, Latino staff thus deployed strategies ranging from self-conscious labeling to politically motivated discourses to insert ethnicity as an element of everyday life into the programs. These strategies had in common a certain transparency and purposefulness of action that embodied the concreteness with which staff constructed ethnicity.

Other strategies, especially in more strongly clinical situations, were more indirect and illustrate how staff conceived the relationship between ethnicity and the clinical:

> According to Helena [psychologist], a major objective of the [Latino] ward is to provide treatment "sensitive" to the patients as well as a learning experience to their relatives. . . . In group therapy sessions, which are conducted in Spanish, patients express to each other and to staff members their ideas as to what is wrong with them and what can be done about it. In the session last Friday, at least two patients related their illness to the existence of "spirits." [These patients], one diagnosed as manic-depressive, expressed to Helena that they were constantly accosted and followed by evil spirits of dead people. One patient attempted to cope with this through prayer; since the spirits are evil and God the antithesis of evil, then He can be relied upon to send them away.
>
> While Helena would not tell the patients that their explanations were wrong, she would offer her own interpretation of them. In the case of spirits, the explanation she conveyed to them and tried to link with their own was that the spirits represented various intensities of depression and that fighting off spirits was psychologically equivalent to attempting to avoid severe depression from overcoming them. *Cultural explanations, according to Helena, are really psychological in nature*; nevertheless, these explanations are important in that they can be used (as in the case of the spirits) to help patients understand themselves better. . . .
>
> I asked her about the usefulness of bringing in an *espiritista* [ritual specialist] in this case and she nearly laughed.

Patients in the programs produced culturally grounded interpretations of their conditions; some merged psychiatric interpretations with "folk" models to render a compound explanatory frame for their illness, while others adhered to a single causal model. Staff at the program consistently translated these interpretations into a psychiatric discourse. The semantic gaps that were to be conciliated by developing culturally sensitive modalities of care thus remained:

> [In a group therapy session,] Victor [psychologist] asked the patients if they believed in witchcraft. One of the patients stated that she believes in God and that one must have faith in order to keep the evil spirits away. Another patient

said that there are two kinds of witchcraft, *"la brujería negra y la brujería blanca /* black witchcraft and white witchcraft"; white witchcraft can financially break people but black witchcraft kills. The patient added that he reads the Bible to keep evil spirits away. . . .

Victor said that in the Middle Ages psychiatric and epileptic patients were thought to be possessed by demons and killed because people didn't know much about mental illness. Even nowadays, some of us [Hispanics] think that mental illness is caused by witchcraft and spirits but modern science had taught us that mental illness is either organic or psychological. . . . The patients assured him that witchcraft exists but they're not that sure that they're *"endemoniados*/bewitched"; they agreed that God is the only one who can cure their illness and if they have faith they'll be able to live normal lives again.

The belief in *espiritismo* is commonplace in Puerto Rico and tightly woven into its cultural fabric; other systems of religious belief are equally intertwined in the culture of other Hispanic groups. Hispanic staff were obviously conscious of these beliefs, but their attitude toward them and to their place in psychiatric care was often determined by occupation and class:

Rosa [TA] mentioned that the training she liked was the one on cultural issues. This training helped her become more sensitive to Hispanic patients and [their] beliefs in *espiritismo* . . . "though I already knew a little about it." I asked Rosa where had she learned about *espiritismo*. She told me that she has a brother who's schizophrenic, "according to the doctors because his brain is damaged. He was very slow as a child. He was always jumping around in class so his teachers would tell my mother to take him to a doctor. She finally did and they thought first that he was retarded and placed him in special education." He was diagnosed as schizophrenic when he was almost 30. I asked her if he was institutionalized in Puerto Rico; Rosa answered that her mother doesn't want him to be in any hospitals because they don't give proper care.

"My mother thinks it was the evil eye," Rosa added. "He was the handsomest in the family, with big, light-colored eyes. There was this woman who was our neighbor and she was bad. She dealt in evil. So she kept telling my brother how beautiful and handsome he was until she cast the evil eye on him. My mother took him to several *espiritista* centers and they told her that, indeed, it had been the evil eye. My mother did everything they told her to, you know, ointments, baths, and that kind of stuff, but nothing helped."

I asked Rosa what did she think it had been. She replied, "I don't believe in *espiritismo* but it's possible that it was the evil eye. Evil exists, I just don't believe one should practice it." (translated from Spanish)

This attitude toward *espiritismo*, common among some Puerto Ricans, underscores the prevalence of native skepticism in the culture. Because no single system of interpretation can be so encompassing as to exhaust mean-

ing, the alternative explanatory frame that *espiritismo* represents is not fully discarded. It constitutes a symbolic fund of knowledge that is held available for its potential to provide a framework for the interpretation and understanding of experience. Puerto Ricans may genuinely profess disbelief in *espiritismo* or reject its practices, but the imperfection in all interpretive systems precludes it from being totally forsaken.

Professional staff with similar cultural experiences, though, would reformulate these experiences on the basis of their socialization into a rational disciplinary domain:

> Petra [psychiatrist] said that she had no problems with *espiritismo*. She would not allow an *espiritista* on the ward but if a patient believes that seeing one would make her feel better, she would allow the patient to go during passes [outside the hospital premises]. Petra's grandmother was an *espiritista*. When she was a young girl, she would go to her grandmother's house and people would come and visit. She would see her grandmother change her voice into somebody else's, light candles, and prescribe remedies. Her grandmother believed that Petra's sister would inherit her spiritual powers of seeing and talking to spirits. Before Petra went to college, she would think, "Why my sister and not me?"
>
> Once she went to college and into pre-med, Petra forgot about *espiritismo*. It wasn't until she was in medical school and took a course in parapsychology that she became seriously aware of her childhood experiences. She began to understand better her grandmother's religious beliefs. As a psychiatrist, she isn't supposed to believe in spirits; it wouldn't be professional. But as she left, Petra added, "At a certain point I inherited my grandmother's powers because she can heal people as an *espiritista* but I can heal people as a psychiatrist."

Cultural experience can thus be refracted through the acquisition of certain forms of rationalized knowledge. Both professional and religious knowledge and skills are ideationally structured as analogous resources for remedying human problems. Yet the clinical context and its purposes constrain the use of the religious as standard practice.

The focus on *espiritismo* and *santería* moved some of the staff to revalue the tension between medical and religious knowledge and led them to seek information on "folk" religious practices. Staff in one of the programs requested a session on *espiritismo* and *santería* from the evaluation team's medical anthropology consultant:

> Barbara [psychiatrist] is so interested in *santería* and *espiritismo* that Oprah [program director] and I laughingly agreed that maybe she should be sent to a center to train. Miguel [psychologist], conversely, seems quite skeptical of the matter and holds on to the clinical model. At the end of the session there was

a rather poignant exchange between them. Miguel was talking rather scoffingly about using these "folk" beliefs in therapy; his point was that, no matter what, the clinical model is controlling, and I think I detected some feeling in him that he views these beliefs as pathological, or just as part of the clinical picture. Barbara countered by pointing out that who were they to know. There are many things in the world that the clinical model can't explain, nor all the science in the world. As scientists, they had to recognize that. Even in physical medicine strange, unexplainable, and/or unexpected things happen—cancers disappear, people recover from terminal conditions. If these beliefs illuminate these unknowns and help to cure people, this made them a very powerful tool to use in their therapy. With a rather humble note in her voice, she finished by saying that *that* was the reason why she herself wanted to know. Miguel had no response to offer.

At another of the programs, staff reconciled patients' religious beliefs with the medical model by taking one of their patients to a ritual specialist to be cleansed and divested of a spell cast on her by a former husband. They explained that they were motivated to do so because it was the patient's "obsession" with this spell that was keeping her from discharge; the underlying purpose was thus institutional. In another case, staff at the same program themselves "exorcised" a patient in a ritual they designed for the same institutional purpose. In both these instances, "folk" ritual was applied not as an authorized and independently valid practice, but instrumentally and unofficially.

Staff's propensity for applying a medical frame to patients' actions and manifestations particularly coalesced when they began to conceptualize the relationship between ethnicity and the clinical as a dichotomy: ethnicity and culture were rendered as content, and the clinical was constituted as form, as the organizing and controlling structure that shaped and determined treatment in the programs. At the end of the evaluation period, the director of one of the programs explicitly characterized their value as resting on this dichotomy. The Latino programs were thus reconstituted into projects that were not clinically different from regular programs because the same modalities of treatment were being applied to their patients; only the *content* of the treatment was different because staff in them used "cultural elements" in their application of these modalities:

I told Miguel [psychologist] that we wanted to know how their endeavors to incorporate language and culture into treatment modalities were coming along. He said that staff had embarked on a process to identify what they were doing. He pointed out that the process of identification was "hard to measure and operationalize." This process was informal. It started with staff considering what it meant for themselves to be Hispanic and turned into more formal

deliberations. Staff experiences were "translated" to two ends: (1) to understand what the patient was about; (2) to incorporate this understanding into treatment. From reflecting about themselves, staff moved on to consider experiences which they've had with patients, instances in which cultural themes were salient. Their aim now is to individualize this understanding and develop treatment strategies for each patient. By using cultural knowledge, they "join" [empathize] with the patient and "reframe" her or his perceptions to direct the patient toward "adjustment." I asked Miguel to clarify how they defined adjustment; did this allude to the clinical model? He said that it did. What they are doing is expressing acceptance and tolerance toward a patient's set of cultural beliefs but also exposing the patients, by telling them about it and explaining it to them, to an alternative resource, "another belief available" which is basically the clinical model. I remarked that this sounded to me [like] some sort of "mainstreaming" and Miguel agreed that it was in a sense and "somewhat." They want to direct patients to understand and accept the treatment resources available to them in the ward.

The "content" themes that they've been able to identify were "the usual": family, for example, and its dynamics and roles. . . . Staff are discussing with patients the extent to which their behavior very often responds to "traditional" values. Staff consciously and purposely react to patients' narratives with more "leniency" and "toleration" but also move on to discuss how these patterns of behavior may be inappropriate in American society. For example, a woman patient may relate incidents in her life when her treatment of her children may have amounted even to child abuse, which the patient articulates as protectiveness. Staff will listen to the patient, show that they understand the cultural reasons why the patient may have thought this behavior adequate but explain to her that, in Anglo culture, the model for socializing children does not revolve around notions of respect and deference but around individualism and independence. The aim is to "bring to the awareness of the patient" the cultural differences so that she or he might understand why one cultural model clashes with the other and how this might be an element in the genesis of psychiatric conditions.

If one examines the dichotomy between form and content for its metaphorical entailments, it is evident that in constituting the clinical as form, program staff consequently constituted it as the structuring force that made the psychiatric process coherent for them. In choosing to articulate the relationship between ethnicity and the clinical and their task of producing culturally sensitive modalities of psychiatric care in terms of this dichotomy, staff in the Latino programs contributed to the reproduction of medical primacy.

Conclusion: Medicalizing Ethnicity

In one of my last visits before the evaluation team wrapped up its three-year field research, I talked with the Latina psychiatrist in one of the programs. Reflecting on her experiences, she told me that she had been averse to the notion of cultural sensitivity when she first heard of the attempts to establish the three demonstration programs. She had sincerely doubted the scientific validity of ethnicizing mental health care. When she was offered the position at one of the programs, she was uneasy about accepting it. As far as she was concerned, it entailed positioning herself not as "a professional" but as "a Hispanic psychiatrist" when she liked to think that her education prepared her to treat all kinds of people, not just those she considered "her own." To work in a bilingual, bicultural psychiatric program for Latino patients amounted, in her mind, to identifying herself publicly as "a psychiatrist who only treated Hispanics"; this would limit her professionally. In spite of these qualms, though, she was persuaded by colleagues to accept the position, at least temporarily.

Now, after living through the experience of contributing to the establishment of the Latino programs, she was thoroughly "sold" on the conceptual value of culturally sensitive care and its benefits for Latino patients. Cultural sensitivity, she told me, did *not* entail the alteration of existing modalities of psychiatric treatment, but called for the use of "cultural elements" for the psychiatric purpose of providing quality mental health care to Latinos.

In defining cultural sensitivity in these terms, constituting "culture" as a reservoir with the potential to be tapped in order to sustain standard modalities of psychiatric care, she confirmed for me the trend that I had already

[145]

remarked. As I concluded in the preceding chapter, the Latino professionals in the programs eventually redefined cultural sensitivity as the use of "cultural elements" as content to the structuring form of psychiatric principles and practices. Defining cultural sensitivity in this way, as I have been arguing, rendered culture an adjunct component of objectified clinical practices.

These definitions evoked for me other kinds of theoretical propositions that tend to separate the "messiness" of sociocultural life from a constructed abstract order that becomes the privileged focus of inquiry, such as happens, for one example, in Saussurean linguistics (Crowley 1990). Whorf's (1956) characterization of Standard Average European languages similarly deploys conceptual categories or habits of thought that ostensibly organize experience into uniform containing units, allowing us to objectify it along axes of temporality and spatiality.

In the preceding chapters I have examined the processes that characterized the establishment of the Latino programs and their development as a paradigmatic instance in the medicalization of ethnicity. My core argument is that medicalizing ethnicity as it happened at these programs allowed it to be incorporated into medical discourses and practices as a pathologized element to be monitored and controlled. Program staff targeted the notion of cultural sensitivity as the core animating principle of their enterprise, constructing a clinical focus that paralleled "native" constructs of culture. My arguments throughout this book have mostly been directed toward establishing how ethnicity becomes the object of institutional discourses and is pushed to the foreground of public and private consciousness, to be incorporated as a constituent factor in the public domain of action represented by medical care. In summarizing her experiences in the program as she did, this Latina psychiatrist attested to the way in which an exercise in reorienting public health resources rendered ethnicity an essential component for the reproduction of the very system its inclusion was aimed at transforming.

Whether as advocates or as program staff, Latino professionals and paraprofessionals deployed a major effort to institute these bilingual, bicultural programs. There were significant medical issues behind these projects; they were meant to address perceived inequalities of access to public resources for mental health care and to remedy the deficiencies that Latino patients suffered under such care. But these actions also constituted the exercise of political agency by Latino mental health practitioners: they engaged in a process facilitated by ideological shifts in U.S. society that shape how ethnicity is addressed in public policy.

Within the context of contemporary cultural, social, political, and economic movements in the United States, civic entitlement is predicated on conditions of "otherness," chief among these being ethnicity. For the state

and its dependencies, ethnicity and other such markers of difference render problematic long-standing beliefs about the eventual social integration and equality of diverse sociocultural groups. This is a particularly salient concern in a nation founded on claims to an egalitarian order which dictates that all members of the society be impartially offered equal opportunity and access to institutional means.

By the 1970s, the interests represented by ethnic activists under the leadership of Latino professionals in the mental health field had converged with governmental concerns about de facto inequality in the state's treatment of Latinos. This convergence brought about the constitution of Latinos as a population "at risk," susceptible to mental illness, and deprived of the kind of mental health care it required. This historic instance of differential definition, both cultural and medical, provided the context for institutionalizing the programs, since the Latino professionals who were advocating for them strategically exploited this notion of risk in order to legitimate their claims. Problematizing Latino mental health "proved" that the programs were sorely needed, and that their establishment responded to actual medical and institutional needs as a matter of enlightened and rational medical and institutional policies and practices, rather than to local identity politics.

Yet, in order to problematize health conditions among Latinos, largely mythic notions and standards of normality were applied; ideationally, the "cultural" and the "medical" were both being constructed as homogeneous, monolithic entities. The process that ensued in these programs, as generated and enacted by their Latino staffs, focused on "culture" as the potential pathological locus of therapeutic applications but also, paradoxically, as a source of curative power that would help remedy what was being represented as a problem in public policy. That is, they were constituting culture as illness and also as cure—the paradox I noted in the introduction as underpinning the medicalization of ethnicity. In articulating culture in these terms, they rendered "culture" and ethnicity as medicalized domains of action.

In the field of relations that the programs represented—with their intersecting occupational, institutional, and ethnic hierarchies—these convergences constituted ethnicity as a subject to be monitored and assessed for its therapeutic possibilities and implications. Staff in the programs embarked on carrying out their mandate to conciliate ethnicity with existing psychiatric practices. They implemented the programs in an evolutionary arc that would begin with instituting Spanish as the official language of everyday as well as therapeutic interactions among staff and patients, continue with the ethnicization of the clinical environment, and, they hoped, culminate in the development of culturally sensitive modes of psychiatric care.

In examining this process, my main purpose has been to focus on the ways in which ethnicity was being constructed in this particular domain of

action. This is a study of ethnicity as it is constructed not among a group of "generic" Latinos or a situated Latino community, but among a specialized occupational group whose members were generating a series of cultural representations for specific instrumental and conceptual purposes. The Latino professionals and paraprofessionals strategically produced and reproduced representations about Latino culture that would converge within the political and institutional contexts in which they were engaged. For one thing, the profile of Latino-ness they produced was directed to underscore features that would set Latinos apart from other major ethnic groups in the United States. For another, this profile incorporated and foregrounded attributes commensurate with prime psychiatric domains of action. By drawing on conventionalized features assumed to be common constituents of a generic Latino cultural type—warmth, docility, personalism, traditionality—these professionals were stereotyping themselves as well as their patients. But this does not necessarily mean that the creation of Latino ethnicity in such a way was either mere artifice or downright insensitivity or stupidity. The generation of contrasting definitional and behavioral cultural profiles under conditions of interethnic contact is essential to the maintenance of boundaries that contribute to the reproduction of modes of identity that mark one ethnic group from another.

These Latino mental health practitioners were applying and exploiting a common cultural practice by which we all engage in reading signs of ethnicity, class, gender, and other distinguishing sociocultural attributes in others. We do so through an accrued stock of types in general circulation, produced in interethnic contact through mutual assessment and contrast.[1] The exercise in ethnic definition these Latinos were engaged in was further legitimated by the need to institute a Latino presence within New York's medical, political, and institutional hierarchies—precisely because the Latino presence has acquired weight and stability as an important component of the city's multicultural and multilingual character.

Stressing a legitimating contrast was thus a controlling strategy in the production of a Latino identity that revolved around affective attributes as the quintessential mark of Latino behavioral and interactional modes. This focus on the affective countered the dehumanizing effects that Latino professionals attributed to the medical setting, the institutional environment, and the host culture itself, which presumably were having such a negative impact on Latinos. But to consummate the process of legitimation, this constructed ethnicity had to be further validated through its incorporation into mainstream psychiatric practices. While ethnicity in American culture has been described as a matter of ascription for its material and symbolic values rather than of content (Sollors 1986), content was reworked into the fabric of ethnic representations in the Latino programs as the field in which ther-

apeutic techniques were to be applied or the subject on which they would be imposed. Ethnicity was thus subordinated to the operations of medical rationality.

The subjection of the self and the emotions under the rationality of institutional power is intrinsic to medical practices in general and psychiatry in particular (Weber 1946; Foucault 1965, 1977, 1978, 1980; Turner 1984). Ironically, from the mechanistic perspective of biomedicine, psychiatry is rendered marginal precisely because it deals with the "untreatable," "soft" dimensions of the psyche—the vagaries of mind and behavior, personal and social, that are construed as deviant—rather than with the material signs that disease inscribes on the physical body (see Johnson 1985:273–74). It is precisely because psychiatry, among the medical disciplines, most explicitly intersects with the cultural and the social that it becomes ever more problematic and liminal to mainstream medical ideology and practices (Romanucci-Ross, Moermann, and Tancredi 1991:259).[2]

But psychiatry is also in a prime position to exert its power on the conceptions of the self, behavior, and interactional styles that constitute both private and public manifestations of ethnicity. Beyond any immediate institutional or medical consequences that it might effect, the application of psychiatric categories generates judgmental assessments that carry moral entailments. Given the "softness" that is often attributed to the field, psychiatric practitioners feel a need for self-legitimation by systematizing psychiatric interpretations and definitions. That is, psychiatry strives for the same rationalization, systematization, and objectification that presumably typify "real" science.[3] It stands in a liminal position by which it implicates the social yet must address the need for achieving a validating rationality.

Conceptually and in practice, the Latino professionals in the programs began to think about culture and ethnicity as content and to treat their patients by instilling in them "rational" modes of behavior as defined under the culturally determined standards of normality embodied in psychiatric models. By engaging in a comparative exercise that did not address—much less transcend—the cultural specificity of psychiatric definitional grids, Latino program staff gauged their patients' behavior, beliefs, and interactional styles against normative psychiatric models that traffic in universal types.

In order to "cure" their patients, the Latino professionals became engaged in tracking ethnic dimensions of behavior that could be scrutinized for their dissonance in relation to mainstream beliefs and practices. The task of reconciling ethnicity with psychiatric modalities of care to produce novel models and practices was operationalized in the patients themselves as a matter of individual choice rather than through these modalities.

Treating their Latino patients became a matter, for program staff, of so-

cializing them into choosing between two sets of culturally prescribed attitudes and behaviors: the Latino set, which retained its pathologizing effect because it was seen as disabling in the host culture, and the psychiatric set, amenable to medication and thus representing the route to a healthy, rational alternative. Staff at the programs predicated mental recovery on the basis of a patient's choosing the normality valued in the host culture over modes of Latino behavior. In this sense, Latino program staff were reproducing the marginal position of Latino culture in U.S. society and contributing to its further subjugation rather than revaluing and empowering it.

The paradoxes and tensions involved in the process I have examined here emerged from contradictions that obtain in a number of sociocultural dimensions and domains: between the maintenance of ethnicity and assimilation, between ethnic resistance and divestment, between cultural and medical practices, between notions of rationality and irrationality. Steinberg (1989:73–74) points out that there is a structural Catch-22 in the history of ethnic groups in the United States. Ethnic revival movements face the dilemma of either being assimilated into the host culture or restoring and maintaining ethnic culture as is apparently authorized by multiculturalist trends. In the first instance, they strain the links between themselves and their own ethnic past; in the second, they become alienated from mainstream U.S. culture and are thus placed in the risky position of reproducing their own disempowerment as "outsiders." The structures of identity still favor monolithic cultural definitions predicated on a modulated and sanitized "American" ethnic model. In spite of the persistence of multiculturalist claims and the establishment, in a variety of sociocultural domains, of services and institutions ostensibly designed to foster cultural maintenance, I would argue that this conundrum still stands, and that processes of ethnic construction remain among the most excruciatingly contested in the United States.

Beyond the constraints of the larger context of U.S. society, within the specific institutional one in which the process of developing the Latino programs occurred, staff's range of action was further conditioned by the dominant ideologies and practices of medical culture. To restore their Latino patients to health, these professionals felt compelled to assimilate them into the medical model sustaining the culture into which they themselves had been occupationally socialized.

These processes, I would suggest, offer no opportunity for closure—however much they may be represented as amenable to completion, or exhaustion, by the existing sociocultural order. Dominant ideologies and public policy in the United States are very much informed by a strong, future-oriented, evolutionistic strain that is historically discernible in movements such as religious revivalism, utopianism, and progressivism. Through them

the nation holds to an ideology of repair and resolution that masks the actual processes of sociocultural reproduction that characterize U.S. society. Thus, closure to contemporary ethno-racial struggles has often been claimed through the institution of leveling policy measures generated during the 1960s civil rights era. Less often addressed are the slippages between these policies and actual practices, or between the institutional measures and the entrenched racializing ideologies that condition them.

My analysis of these processes as they obtained in the Latino programs was determined by the conditions under which I learned about them. That is, since my project, however it eventually diverged, began with their evaluation, it was staff that we evaluators focused on. This gave me the opportunity to examine an instance in which ethnic elites exploit their advantageous position in the best of faith but generate paradoxical results and unintended consequences.

As I pointed out in the introduction, here and there in my work there are glimpses of the individuals on whose minds and bodies the therapeutic process was being applied. In the utilitarian terms used in the programs and measured by such indices as discharge rates, treatment needs, and the achievement of institutional privileges, the Latino patients in the programs "improved": their induction into the programs appeared to alleviate mental illness for some, even though many were not discharged and others relapsed.

I always suspected that patients improved because they learned, as I suggested in the introduction, to make it both crazy and ethnic and manipulate their own condition of patienthood, rather than because "culture" is imbued with *intrinsic* curative power. To agree with such a characterization of culture would oversimplify the concept. Patients in the Latino programs engaged in cunning strategies of accommodation to the objectifying terms of medical culture and treatment, even when these strategies required them to play to the hilt their subordinated and dependent role. They demonstrated their ability to exploit institutional conditions that differed from their previous experiences in other clinical spaces—precisely because these conditions allowed them to engage in overt displays of ethnicity, to enact Latino-ness and foreignness in order to capitalize on the existing orders of entitlement that value such demonstrations.

I do not think that success within the instrumental terms of institutional culture defeats my argument that the process in which these patients were involved was objectifying. That the patients improved only attests to their own habituation to their institutionalization rather than to some sort of autonomous curative effect wrought by the insertion of terms of ethnicity that were themselves co-opted by the institutional and medical discourses prevalent in the programs.

Addressing primordialism as a subtext in processes of identity construction, Wilmsen (1996:2–3) argues:

> [P]rimordialism cannot help but be a subtext—for ethnicity as an existential presence is founded on just one premise: the conviction of the reality of endemic cultural and social, often racial, difference. The premise is faulty, but if phenomena are real in their effects, they are real; this is the power of primordial arguments. The obverse is that they must be addressed as real. Such conviction is not confined to the everyday world of the ethnenes, the subjects of ethnicity; it is common in the highest academic towers. . . .
>
> Historical deconstruction certainly robs ethnicity of the mythic sense of timelessness on which it thrives, but to say that ethnicity is artificially constructed does not give us license to dismiss it as illegitimate. Dismissal only begs the question of how far back in time we have to go in order to satisfy criteria of "genuineness." The intellectual and political task, therefore, is to find a vocabulary that embraces forms of ethnic identification that are flexible and polyvalent rather than only those which are exclusivistic and chauvinistic. . . . Primordialist ethnic claims are nothing more than claims to ownership of the past and rights to its use for present purposes.

Wilmsen thus repositions primordialism as a crucial subtext for its rootedness in a very basic belief—that cultural difference exists—shared across sociocultural domains. (This is, after all, precisely the ultimate anthropological principle.) As I see it, primordialism encompasses and operates through the kinds of essentializing strategies that I have documented in the Latino programs.

If we presuppose primordialism as an actual force in ethnicity, what happened at the Latino programs was neither unexpected nor necessarily that unusual. What I have documented and argued here is that the Latino mental health practitioners were engaged in an essentializing—and, thus, primordializing—strategy by reasserting difference as a major sociocultural marker of both identity and experience. Whether this exercise in identity construction was (or could be) "successful" in the sense of achieving what was being pursued is not the best measure of its merits. Its meaning lies elsewhere than in such pragmatics. However objectifying and however much it contributed to reproducing and reconstituting subordination, I would suggest, it is still important to remember that these Latino practitioners engaged in essentializing Latino culture and Latino identity for the purpose, as Wilmsen would argue, of claiming and using the past to address very pressing contemporary issues and conditions.

Notes

Introduction

1. I follow what has become common cross-disciplinary use by drawing from Foucault's (1972) notion of discourse. "Discourse" refers to the application of language to carve out specialized fields of knowledge that are historically and socially located yet acquire a universal and ahistoric character. Though we think of discourses as coherent and unifying, they are actually complex, paradoxical ways of talking about events, things, relations, and subjects. Discourses position those who use them and that to which they are applied within specific social fields and hierarchies. Understood in this sense, discourse becomes a productive notion for examining sociocultural processes in institutional settings marked by unequal power relations. My use of the concept of "institution" is informed by Bourdieu's (1977, 1991), since I see it not in the traditional social science sense as an organized, structured, collectivizing entity that exercises a specialized social function, but as "a relatively durable set of social relations which *endows* individuals with power, status and resources of various kinds" (Thompson 1991: 8). I also follow Bourdieu (1977, 1990) in articulating the relationship between discourse and practice into "a logic of practice" that makes them mutually constitutive. I have been strongly influenced by scholarship that explores the linkages between language and cultural context (e.g., Ochs 1988; Schieffelin 1990), especially in everyday practices. These theoretical elaborations share the idea that sociocultural actors draw from and apply culturally prescribed knowledge through the structured and structuring capacities of discourse and practice. This is what allows all members of a culture with the same ideational sets of beliefs and behaviors to exploit various material and symbolic resources. These notions may sometimes seem overdetermining, but I believe they also capture best the complexities that characterized the Latino programs I examine—and other sociocultural phenomena, for that matter.

2. The people who worked in these programs designated themselves, the programs, and their patients as "Hispanic[s]," and I am bound to honor their practice. "Latino," however, has become the general term of choice, to the point where I believe it is on the verge of the institutional co-optation that "Hispanic" suffered. Yet both remain contested. As Oboler (1995) points out, debates over the adequacies of the labels have ultimately become something of a red herring embodying the potentially enervating effects of reductionism, reification, and di-

visions among the nation's complex Latino constituencies. Di Leonardo (1984) addresses labeling as a process of mutual identity construction which has its uses, but equally argues that ethnicity cannot be reduced to labeling. As I have pointed out elsewhere (1996:4), labeling implicates issues of specification and homogenization, but also of power, resistance, and agency. Although national origin remains the favored identifier, as is sustained by other data sets (e.g., de la Garza et al. 1992), I use both "Latino" and "Hispanic" in this book, recognizing that the use of either umbrella term is situational and strategic. I retain the use of "Hispanic" whenever I draw, through direct quotation or in paraphrase, from the data collected at the programs and where I "voice"—in Bakhtinian terms—the people in them. Otherwise, I use "Latino" as the general designator.

3. I use the terms "clinical" and "medical" interchangeably. The programs were mostly designed for inpatient care, and the clinical setting, as I explain, was important for the purposes of validating cultural sensitivity, since it gave the Latino practitioners in the program the opportunity to develop culturally sensitive practices within the totality of conditions that inpatient care represents.

4. Di Leonardo (1998) argues that contemporary anthropological practices continue to efface issues of unequal power relations within the United States, particularly with regard to women and ethnic communities. I share her concerns about this blind spot in U.S. anthropology when it continues to define itself as the field of inquiry that focuses on "difference" while casting itself and U.S. society in the role of unmarked and deculturated normative center (in spite of a long-standing Americanist tradition, as well as the articulation of the anthropological enterprise, *à la* Mead, as a venue for perpetuating the nation's self-understandings). As di Leonardo points out, anthropologists have contributed to the production and reproduction of entwined "noble" and "nasty" savages in both the scholarly and the popular imagination by exoticizing "others," be they foreign or local. The dichotomy of evil and good that marks di Leonardo's entwined savages correlates with and is reiterated in my examination of the uses of culture within psychiatric domains in which it is paradoxically constituted both as illness and as cure.

Chapter 1 *"It sounds like Hispanics stereotyping other Hispanics!"*

1. I use pseudonyms for persons, places, and organizations throughout this book, except for the two state agencies that oversaw the programs—the New York State Office of Mental Health and New York City's Health and Hospital Corporation.

2. Bourdieu's (1977) well-known notion of habitus encompasses sets of dispositions that we incorporate into our consciousness and that structure our everyday actions and perceptions. Habitus is culturally constructed, shared, and transmitted; because it is both structured and structuring, it contributes to the reproduction of cultural norms, principles, practices, even itself. It thus shapes our sociocultural practices but is itself shaped by them. As I see it, habitus bridges the gaps between structural conditions and what people actually do within the strictures that these conditions establish, thus eroding the deterministic sense that the notion of structure carries and retaining a sense of human agency. See also Giddens (1979).

3. The American Psychiatric Association (APA) work group that produced the contemporary version of the *Diagnostic and Statistical Manual of Psychiatric Disorders*, Third Edition—Revised (1987), or *DSM III-R*, expressed similar concerns in an introductory note urging caution in the application of its classificatory grid to people from "other" ethnic and cultural groups (APA 1987:xxvi). When the APA began to revise the manual to produce the *DSM-IV* (1994), it considered adding to it a "cultural axis." In *DSM* discourse, an "axis" is a particular domain of information, articulated in terms of the mental disorders and medical conditions, psychosocial and environmental problems, and functional levels exhibited by the person being diagnosed and treated. The "multiaxial" approach that the APA advocates in the

manual promotes the application of a holistic "biopsychosocial" model in subjecting the person to the totalizing effects of the grid (APA 1994:25ff.) According to the expanded section "Ethnic and Cultural Considerations" in *DSM-IV* (APA 1994:xxiv), the "solution" was to replace the previous cautionary warning by noting existing or already identified "cultural variations" relevant to each classification, adding an appendix describing "culture-bound" syndromes, and designing and attaching an outline for "cultural formulations" to guide practitioners in evaluating and reporting the impact of an individual's "cultural context."

4. Cohn (1987) discusses a similar experience in which "speaking" the language of a specialized disciplinary and occupational domain contributes to its ideological reproduction. Learning to speak the language inducts one into such domains' modes of thought, their particular world view and ethos (Geertz 1973), or habitus (Bourdieu 1977).

5. This methodological tension is an issue that I do not address here as thoroughly as it deserves or I would wish, although I touch on it in passing. It generated much friction and debate among evaluators, program staff, and bureaucrats, all of whom represented an array of disciplinary and practical knowledge.

6. These included the chairs of the programs' advisory boards and the president of the local organization of Latino mental health practitioners which had advocated for the establishment of the programs. See chapter 2.

7. Cf. Merry (1990), who uses the term "legal consciousness" to articulate the ways in which people understand and use the legal system. Of course, I claim no originality for "ethnic consciousness." The term is a common expression in popular use, part and parcel of a generalized discourse on cultural pluralism prevalent in contemporary U.S. society. In its "popular" sense it marks people's awareness of their own ethnic roots and is often mobilized for political purposes of empowerment under a quantifying rationale: that raising ethnic consciousness among individuals will translate into a commonality of interest and political purpose for the collective good of all—the more consciousness, the more power. This form of "ethnic consciousness," as popularly used, is subsumed under what I mean by "ethnic consciousness," which encompasses broader, and even contradictory, ranges of thought and action in order to stress complexity and depth of understanding. In my sense, then, devaluing ethnicity as a hindrance to political, social, and economic mobility and advocating for ethnic divestment would be just as much a manifestation of ethnic consciousness as the other kind. In the case at hand, as I argue in the text, ethnic consciousness is configured as a bounded, static, portable form of knowledge.

8. The 1970s "ethnic revival" in the United States (and its celebration) became a reaffirmation of "white" ethnicity, obscuring the pervasive marginalization of historically racialized groups and reconstituting prevailing ethno-racial hierarchies. The acclamation surrounding an unproblematic "multiculturalism" which became the dominant national self-definitional strategy further contributed to marking members of racialized and marginalized ethnicities as intrinsic losers when the alleged shift to cultural plurality did not translate into structural advancement for them. Thus, in accordance with Steinberg (1989), Omi and Winant (1991), and Urciuoli (1996), although I have adopted "ethnicity" here, this does not mean that I hold all "ethnicities" equal—because the racialized identity order in the United States does not.

9. Blu (1979) points out that the biologization and "naturalization" of cultural difference entailed in the production of phenotypical racial categories, as historically happens in the United States, has moral overtones. Ethnic categories, perceived as categories "in culture," presuppose the existence of a community that provides individual members with a sustaining collective moral order, place, and authority; racial categories, understood as categories "in nature," are viewed as devoid of any such communal moral presence and dimensions. She is generating not abstractions but empirically based generalizations, as exemplified in the historic tendency among Latino communities to avoid their own racialization in the United States by opting for "cultural" or "national" designations as terms of identity, for example, "Hispanic" "Hispano," "Latino," "Puerto Rican," "Mexican American," "Chicano," and so on. See de León

(1983), Rodríguez (1991), Gutiérrez (1995), Oboler (1995), Rodríguez and Sánchez-Korrol (1996), among others. Blu's arguments and the predominance of national and hyphenated identities articulate very well with Urciuoli's (1996) notions of "ethnicizing" and "racializing" discourses, which I discuss in the text.

10. I am reminded of this point quite frequently in relation to yet another common socio-cultural descriptor in the United States: the sociological quantification of identity as "minority." Newspaper headlines often proclaim something or the other about "minorities"; one reads the text to discover that it addresses only African Americans and has nothing to do with Latinos, Asian Americans, or Native Americans (or with women, who are also frequently subsumed under the minority rubric). This is yet another form of colonization endured by Latinos and other groups in the United States: the erasure, within the polarized racial dichotomy, of the specificities of the politics of identity in which they are embedded. The metaphorical entailment in the term "minority" itself indicates how groups are perceived and located in the existing hierarchies of power.

11. Contemporary with the establishment of the Latino programs, this extensive body of works includes Haberman (1976), Karno (1966), Levine and Padilla (1980), Malgady, Rogler, and Costantino (1987), Malzberg (1965), Padilla and Ruíz (1973), Price and Cuellar (1981), Rosado (1980), and Vázquez (1982), among others. The *Hispanic Journal of Behavioral Sciences* addresses issues of mental health.

Chapter 2 Negotiating Ethnicity

1. While the analysis and interpretation of the place of this report in the imagination of the Latino mental health professionals involved in the programs is my own, I must acknowledge that it was engendered by Lessinger's (1991) account of the document both as an official expression in the movement to improve the delivery of mental health services for Latinos and as a contextual factor in the subsequent attempts to institutionalize programs and practices that were directed to address the issue.

2. I omit the extensive and unwieldy citations from this report to make it readable; like so many government reports (and dissertation literature reviews), it cites every conceivable source, and should be consulted directly by those interested in that level of detail. My focus here is on the statements of the report itself.

3. During my fieldwork, the CHMH performed crisis intervention in two major disasters in the New York City area that affected mostly (if not entirely) Latinos: the Happy Land nightclub fire and the Avianca plane crash. The Happy Land fire was caused by a disgruntled suitor who set fire to a neighborhood club in the Bronx, a case of arson in which eighty-seven patrons died. Seventy-two persons died in the Avianca disaster when, on a flight from Colombia, a plane ran out of fuel and crashed on Long Island. Staff from the Plymouth program provided aid to victims and relatives, a gesture that garnered the program great community support, underscored the need for trained bilingual personnel in such emergencies, and contributed to the program's institutional prestige and local legitimacy.

4. Developments in ethnic movements and the fragmentation attendant widespread assertions of cultural difference in the United States have obviously diminished the force of this argument. Contemporary movements for the establishment of exclusive educational facilities for particular ethnic groups and other such quasi-ethnocentric manifestations of ethnic power that draw their persuasiveness and legitimacy from the cultural currency of "multiculturalism" indicate as much. The establishment of the Latino programs is obviously an outgrowth of these decentering responses to broader issues of power, hegemony, knowledge, and identity.

5. Senior staff at Plymouth's Latino program shared with us work histories of rising through the ranks from custodial positions to supervisory ones. The first director of the program was himself a second-generation Plymouth employee whose Puerto Rican father had

migrated to the area in the 1940s to work at Plymouth; the director himself began in a nursing position, rising to become a mid-level administrator.

6. A full exploration of the debate about the biological ("natural") versus the social basis for language acquisition is beyond the scope of this book. For a brief statement of the debate at the time, still ongoing, see Ochs and Schieffelin (1984). Representations about language in the Latino programs sounded to me quite close to Chomskian theorizing: "In the case of language the language faculty, a physical mechanism in the sense already explained [i.e., as part of the natural material world], has certain definite properties, not others. These are the properties that the theory of universal grammar seeks to formulate and describe. These properties permit the human mind to acquire a language of a specific type, as we have seen. The same properties exclude other possible languages as 'unlearnable' by the language faculty" (Chomsky 1988:149).

7. The proposal was for two, rather than the eventual three, because at this point CHMH was negotiating only with OMH, and what was being envisioned was the official establishment of the Plymouth program and one other at a state facility with a different institutional setting and population profile for comparative purposes. The city and HHC had not yet become fully involved in the negotiations. See chapter 3.

8. They also argue that Latino communities are constituted as consumers by corporate capitalism, but this basis for identity predication is less germane to my purposes here.

9. I discuss elsewhere the complex issue of the relationship between patient's language, therapist's language, language preference in the expression of psychopathology, and the effects of linguistic dissimilarity on psychiatric therapy. The basic idea that informed the process of institutionalizing the programs, however, is, as expressed in the CHMH proposal, a sort of linguistic regression.

10. The HHI no longer exists.

Chapter 3 Clinical Topographies

1. The other two instances of training activities that I witnessed or found documented in other researchers' notes were suggested by the evaluation team. Both drew on one of the consultants, who, for one, devised a checklist of elements and experiences to record in the patients' medical record in order to elicit more "cultural" details of their life histories, such as language abilities, immigration history, and so on. The second activity involved the lecture on *espiritismo* and *santería* that I draw on in chapter 5 to illustrate how program staff applied certain Latino cultural practices for their therapeutic possibilities.

2. The policy lasted until the late 1940s. The literature on this issue is fairly extensive, but Zentella (1980) provides a succinct synthesis of its vicissitudes and ideological implications; she also schematizes the correlations between language ideologies and policies and the island's history.

3. Though Plymouth had many Latinos on staff, its upper-level administrators were concerned that there were not enough to implement fully the program's staffing needs. This was particularly so in the case of professional staff, since the number of Latinos in the mental health professions declines as one goes up the occupational ladder. Interestingly, though, it was at paraprofessional levels that the programs failed to achieve totally Latino staffing, while managing to staff professional positions almost fully with Latinos. This result shows how energetically professionals were recruited—perpetuating the suspicion that the programs were solely a self-interested scheme for improving the professional labor market for Latinos. Non-Latino paraprofessional staff were used mostly on night and weekend shifts, giving rise to administrative and interactional problems—mostly charges and countercharges about negligent patient care between Latino and non-Latino personnel on the different work shifts.

4. Throughout the course of these legal proceedings, upper-level administrators at Plymouth were confident of prevailing in court. They believed they had made a very strong case for specialized ethnic staffing. They reiterated arguments about the correlation between adequacy of care and outcome-oriented medical and institutional ideologies that place a premium on the curative effects of institutional treatment. They capitalized as well on the ethnically driven public policies that havé produced a discourse of rights and entitlements on the basis of cultural difference.

5. As in the other two programs, non-Latino staff at Plymouth reportedly grumbled about the "special" Latino program. In all three programs, these comments often took one of two kinds of discursive formulas, which I heard frequently in the field and are not uncommon in the United States: "If Hispanics have a ward for themselves, why not a ward for Chinese (Italians, Jews, . . .)?" and "My parents came over without anything and they had to learn the language and get used to being here and no one helped them! Why can't Hispanics?" I think of the first as a statement about equal entitlement and the second as a master migration narrative of assimilation. Both, though, betray an interesting touch of assimilated nativism.

6. A day program is a structured course of activities for higher-functioning patients who are not a security risk to themselves and others and are considered strong candidates for discharge. It is a privilege akin to minimum security in prison systems, and likewise entails a less restrictive setting either outside or within the institutional environment.

7. At the very end of the evaluation period the wards were converted from locked to open wards, meaning that the doors to the wards were open but the doors of the buildings were locked. This measure actually enhanced staff mobility and contributed to improved surveillance.

8. Staff at the program told me that their experiences at the house had led them to suspect it was haunted. Though they were mostly joking, its isolation and old-fashioned look, the appearance of being designed to look lived in though it was not, certainly would have inspired such fantasies.

9. Recidivism was common in all the Latino programs. The psychiatrist at Jefferson once told me that he estimated the number of "revolving door" patients—those who returned or were brought back to the program after discharge—at 80 percent. All of us on the evaluation team often encountered patients at Jefferson who had been discharged from Northern, another index of recidivism. The catchment area of these two programs overlapped, which was not the case with Plymouth's, as it was too distant from the urban facilities. Another indication of recidivism was the extensive history of intermittent institutionalization in the medical records of middle-aged and elderly patients. I do not know whether other facilities also sustain similar high rates of recidivism or if this was unique to the Latino programs, but it was a matter of great concern to their staffs. Conversely, it was a circumstance that could be strategically used to strengthen claims about the lack of quality mental health care for Latinos, the deficiencies of the public care system, or the propensity of Latinos toward mental illness and thus their status as a population at risk. Other mental health officials who were critical of the programs maintained that their conditions actually fostered institutionalization: patients' normal tendencies toward institutional dependency were heightened by the ethnically sensitive character of the programs. This was often presented as one of the reasons for lagging discharge rates. More hostile was the interpretation of a non-Latino administrator and psychiatrist at Jefferson who charged that staff misunderstood cultural sensitivity to mean that they should "coddle" patients, making for low discharge rates and rendering the concept of cultural sensitivity clinically and bureaucratically suspect.

10. I discuss the ramifications this designation had on the institutional politics of identity at Jefferson and its effects on the process of ethnic definition in the chapters that follow.

11. At the end of the evaluation, in the programs' third and final year as pilot projects, Dr. Ramírez, the Colombian psychiatrist who was CHMH's president when the programs were first proposed, was appointed director of the psychiatry department at Jefferson. The change

was expected to improve the administrative situation, and there were initial signs that it was effective. Interestingly, he had raised the issue of Jefferson's administrative ambiguities and anticipated the problems these could generate with the then-director of psychiatry at Jefferson, an African American. The latter acknowledged the situation and told Dr. Ramírez that these problems would eventually be solved because a Latino would be appointed to direct the psychiatry department.

12. Staff at the Plymouth day program were best able to arrange for the regular availability of such foods for their patients. This underscored the day program's special character as compared with the ward, where patients had only regular institutional food on an everyday basis.

13. This notwithstanding the programs' requirement that mandated training in cultural sensitivity for Latino staff.

Chapter 4 The "Mother Tongue" and the "Hispanic Character"

1. Rodríguez (1991), although addressing only the case of Puerto Ricans, offers a good synthesis of the economic and social displacements that immigrant or "minority" groups have suffered in New York City since the 1960s. Takaki (1990) also summarizes the situation of Puerto Ricans and discusses that of other Latino groups as well as other racialized "minorities" in the nation, in the context of his notion of the "fourth iron cage," which indexes capitalist development in the United States and differentially positions ethno-racial communities.

2. These numbers were compiled by the New York Department of City Planning (1990) on the basis of the 1990 national census, with the caveat that they were subject to correction for undercount or overcount. Although the numbers may not exactly reflect demographic "reality," the slippage in counting is not likely to alter substantially the percentages of change for any of the groups, or the trends of increase and decrease that the original numbers indicate, and on which the Latino professionals who advocated for the programs based their numbers argument.

3. The issue of the undercount survived throughout the decade, triggering litigation and legislation. The role of the census as a redistributive mechanism organizing political entitlement for the allocation of public resources is apparent when one considers that the 1990 census, with its alleged undercount, was not challenged just by activist elites within the identifiable populations whose claims had been undermined. It generated coalitions of states, cities, and urban counties which mobilized in the courts; redistribution, after all, benefits those in the "middle" as much as, even more than, its intended recipients. In the Manhattan federal district court, one coalition filed suit seeking to require the Department of Commerce to approve an adjustment to the census after the Bush administration (1988–92) decided against correcting the undercount. The adjustment would have resulted in an additional $1 billion in federal aid to urban areas on the basis of corrected population counts. An expert witness for the plaintiffs—Eugene Ericksen, a professor of sociology and statistics and census adviser to the Department of Commerce—testified at the trial that, in spite of the department's attempts to improve its counting procedures, the 1990 census showed a substantial undercount of minority groups, particularly African Americans and Latinos (*New York Times*, May 13, 1992). The undercount was allegedly due to the problems census takers face in counting the urban poor, presumably owing to lack of access, the number of homeless, undocumented migrants, and so on. The correlation of poverty, homelessness, and other such marginalizing social conditions with ethno-racial difference is significant for what it says about the differential structural positioning of these "minorities" in the national hierarchy.

The debates over the census took on ever more explicit and telling—yet not totally unexpected—political consequences. The Bureau of the Census, in order to cure the problem of undercounting, developed an alternate method to the traditional headcount in which statistical sampling would be used to estimate the size and characteristics of local populations (*New York Times*, June 7, 1998). This generated a scramble among members of Congress, especially

those whose districts stand to lose if the counts of "minorities" are revised upward as a result. In 1999, when the Clinton administration's proposal to apply sampling in the 2000 census was legally challenged, the Supreme Court ruled against sampling on constitutional grounds.

4. Woolard's work on bilingualism in Catalonia challenges facile assumptions about the correlation among different hierarchical orders. She documents how a national language (Spanish) can accrue less symbolic capital than a regional one (Catalonian) despite its position as a homogenizing language whose institutionalization pursues hegemonic goals. Her work underscores the importance of examining the specifics of different historical situations and structural relations in order to ascertain the significance of various sets of linguistic ideologies and practices in multilingual communities.

5. There are, of course, continuities between these contemporary versions and long-standing nativist strains. See Higham (1963); Steinberg (1989); Takaki (1990).

6. The sociolinguistic literature on language and Latino communities in the United States grew markedly during the 1970s. After a relative lapse in production in the 1980s, it appears to be growing again. Representative authors, articles, and anthologies include Fishman et al. (1971); Durán (1981); Amastae and Elías-Olivares (1982); Sánchez 1983 [1994]; Ramírez (1988); Zentella (1980, 1990a, 1990b); Urciuoli (1991). Silva-Corvalán (1994), Urciuoli (1996), Torres (1997), and Zentella (1997) represent more recent scholarship on the topic; although these scholars come from somewhat different disciplinary backgrounds, to varying degrees and effects their work is informed by an ethnographic perspective. This is not an exhaustive list, but will serve to orient interested readers.

7. Although the focus in the literature was on language, culture is the silent premise that informs it. Cultural and racial mismatch had also become a concern in psychiatric and psychological practice, with some practitioners arguing that white therapists could not effectively treat ethno-racially diverse patients. These concerns are embedded in a history of interethnic relations permeated with racism and a product of the ethnic activism and civil rights movements that characterized the 1960s and early 1970s.

Sue (1988) critiques that assumption, arguing that the concern was being misconceptualized, because the empirical problem of effectiveness had been confounded with moral and ethical issues produced by sociopolitical conditions. He suggests that ethnicity by itself could not be the determining factor in the effectiveness of therapeutic outcomes since one can expect variation in the range of individual values, experiences, and behaviors that a culture can accommodate. Sue advocates for an individual-centered approach and considers ethnicity "a distal factor" in therapeutic outcomes, even while urging further research on the issue of cultural mismatch in psychiatric practices as an empirical problem. I cite this particular article because, at the time of my fieldwork, researchers in the field considered it a seminal work in the body of literature that treated the issue of mismatch and the relevance of cultural and linguistic difference in psychiatry and psychology. It was thus used in the analysis of issues pertaining to the development of the programs during their evaluation, and would shape program staff formulations when we elicited feedback. I still find Sue's stance problematic, as I did then. In practice, it tends to excise the effects of culture on an individual's life and, in a sense, begs the question of mismatch even while recognizing the tensions inherent in ethno-racial hierarchies in the United States. It reproduces the universalistic and individualistic ethos that governs biomedicine in general, and psychology in particular, as products of a western European ideology that "generally locate[s] the causes of disorder in individual minds, personalities, and neuroanatomies" (Marsella and White 1982:5).

8. Malgady, Rogler, and Costantino (1987) summarize the research as it stood then. I should add that if I sound tentative about the researchers' language model, it is because I was never explicit about whether they were actually considering one and, if so, exactly what it was. Thus the force of the language habitus: it seemed to me that the very idea of a model of language, its use in communication and expression, and its place in the constitution of sociocultural agency were enigmatic, nonexistent, or unexamined issues to those who were probing the notion of mismatch.

9. The phenomenon is not exclusive to Latino communities in the Northeast but has been extensively documented among Mexican American/Chicano communities of the West and the Southwest for several decades. Immigrating nationals from other Spanish-speaking countries exhibit similar code-switching behavior to that documented in long-standing Puerto Rican and Chicano communities. See note 6.

10. This is not to say that I am challenging its truthfulness and legitimacy. I am simply underscoring how the event was shaped in the framework of a particular narrative genre, and applied as a symbolic template to assign meaning to the effects of cultural and linguistic difference within clinical settings.

11. One is reminded of Whorf's (1956) examination of grammatical categories and his characterization of Standard Average European languages which tend toward objectification, including the constitution of entities as vessels or containers of abstract experiential components.

12. The "distinctiveness" of African American culture is an old debate. See Blauner 1970.

Chapter 5 Occasions of Treatment

1. I treat *espiritismo* and *santería* as a single religious system, after Harwood's (1977) description of them as traditions of spiritism. They are of dissimilar origin—*espiritismo* entered the Latino Caribbean through Europe, while *santería*, generally recognized as being of Cuban origin, is rooted in African religious practices—and embody ideological and ritualistic differences as well. A salient difference between the two is the incorporation of African spirits into the spirit hierarchy in *santería* as opposed to *espiritismo's* assimilation of Christian saints. What underpins my treatment, however, is the syncretistic nature that both practices have acquired in New York City, generating a sort of *santerismo*. Not only do Harwood's (1977:49) fieldwork observations sustain his interpretations along these lines, but also I have witnessed the trend in my personal experiences of Puerto Rican/Latino culture in the city and, most important, in the Latino programs. Although there may be differences and competition between the ritual specialists of each practice, there is much ambiguity and lack of specification among Latino adepts; both *espiritismo* and *santería* are treated as alternative religious resources that are mobilized and ranked together against established religions as well as against other sociotherapeutic systems of signification in the host society, particularly medicine and psychiatry.

2. Harwood (1977) illustrates the interest that had already been generated by the 1970s in drawing upon *santería* and *espiritismo* for psychiatric purposes. See also Ruiz and Langrod (1984). Generally, in New York City, at the time of the establishment of the Latino programs, applying *santería* and *espiritismo* to psychiatric purposes was somewhat more commonplace than many of the professionals in the programs assumed it to be. I always suspected that minimizing previous efforts was another highly constructed argument deployed to validate the programs.

3. The designation of a series of recreational and occupational patient activities as "therapy" has resulted in the professionalization of specific disciplinary domains such as physical therapy, occupational therapy, and even genres such as dance, music, and art therapy. Interestingly, though, the staff who occupied these positions at the programs were generally classified as therapy aides (TA), distinguishable from garden variety mental health therapy aides (MHTA) only by the assignment of special tasks. As far as I could ascertain, none of the front-line staff who actually organized and supervised therapy activities for the patients held advanced degrees in specialized academic fields. Their expertise was more practice-based.

4. Of all staff, nurses were the most likely to be non-Latino and English-monolingual. A general dearth of nurses (at the time a nationwide problem) militated against the successful recruitment of Latinos for the position. The programs usually strove to staff daytime shifts with Latino nurses and assign non-Latinos to night and weekend shifts, when the lack of scheduled activities entailed less contact with patients and so the need for Spanish-speaking

staff was thought to be less pressing. The same schedule was applied to MHTAs, some of whom were also non-Latino and English-monolingual.

5. I am using the term "director" for economy. The actual titles of the people occupying the top position varied.

6. David Dinkins was then New York City's mayor. The situation in the Latino programs document the long-standing ambivalence his term revived between the city's Latino and African American administrators over the allocation of public resources and civic entitlements. Staff at the programs would often speculate about Dinkins's administration in a judgmental gamut that ranged from barely veiled racism, through pragmatic assessments that, after all, everyone looks after his own and that is what politics is about, to manifestations of faith in interethnic solidarity between African Americans and Latinos against a common white, Anglo/Euro-American enemy.

7. The lack of differentiation in address indicates the subordinate position assigned to paraprofessional staff. Professional staff usually enjoyed the honorific professional address (e.g., "doctor") and would be addressed by last name rather than the informal first-name address used with paraprofessionals. Sometimes patients would refer to professional staff as "the psychologist" or "the social worker," using occupational titles that emphasize status.

8. This is not to say, as typified knowledge about Latino cultures has it, that Latinos are more hierarchical, class-bound, and submissive than Anglo-Americans, constituting U.S. culture as more progressive than and morally superior to Latino cultures. On the contrary, along with others, I believe that the cultural history of the United States is characterized by a hegemonic denial of class that masks the structures of inequality prevalent throughout it.

9. These plans also organized outpatient care for those patients who had achieved discharge.

10. Of course, there were also pragmatic reasons in acute cases for appealing to others for information: patients in crisis are generally in no condition to construct a life narrative or explain their situation. This does not negate my argument, however.

11. The issue was more succinctly stated to me as a joke by Philip Merrifield (since deceased), who taught psychology at New York University, when I was a graduate student in the spring of 1989: "How many psychologists does it take to change a light bulb? Just one—but the light bulb must *want* to be changed." Ferrara (1994:23) also includes this joke.

12. In her study of spirit possession among Malay women, Ong (1987) notes how expressions and actions that issue from native systems of belief represent the reconstitution of native values and a manifestation of resistance in institutional settings that are foreign to a local culture.

13. These were often performative strategies animated by a sort of "épater les bourgeois" spirit, as a way of challenging generational claims to authority. This was effected linguistically by code-switching into English and maintaining dominance by controlling the floor, thus imposing a particular symbolic frame of understanding.

14. Patients at the programs often applied the stigmatizing label "crazy" to themselves and their fellow inmates to manipulate everyday situations of authority. They were generally aware of their condition, but they equally set up situational gradations of "craziness," which they could then mobilize to make the most of their institutional situation.

15. This kind of group is designed to educate patients about psychological and psychiatric treatment.

Conclusion

1. This is not to say that I am "naturalizing" these strategies of contrast. It should be evident that what I argue, and have been arguing, is that they are culturally constituted strategies however much they may be cross-culturally drawn upon and applied. And of course these con-

trastive strategies are compounded with others intended to establish each group's participation in a basic sense of humanity.

2. There has been an increasing biologization of psychiatry (and psychology) since I first addressed this issue. I have already discussed the reliance on psychotropic medication in the programs and the dissonance of the practice vis-à-vis the mandate for cultural sensitivity in the Latino programs. I also noted briefly Arthur Kleinman's critique of the biologization of psychiatry which anticipated this turn, and I want to expand these important issues here. Kleinman (1988) noted the orientation in contemporary psychiatry, as it "has undertaken a voyage in the opposite direction," toward the biologization of psychiatric interpretations and practices, which he denounces. Teasing out the sociocultural circumstances that produce an ethos of biologization among psychiatric practitioners, Kleinman writes:

> In spite of evidence pointing to the social origins of depression, the thrust of the research is on the identification of its biological correlates, *even if these are secondary*. Biology has cachet with psychiatrists; anthropology and sociology do not. . . .
>
> There is [in psychiatry] a systematic resistance to dealing with social sources of depression and other psychiatric conditions. . . . In spite of the interest of some psychiatrists and psychologists in social factors and prevention, the orientation of the mental health professions overall contributes to this problem. For psychiatry, the neurosciences hold out the hope of escaping marginality and catching up with the rest of biomedicine . . . ; for psychology, cognitive science and behavioral medicine are the darlings of research funding agencies and hold the promise of financial support for clinical specialists. But the political economy and the cultural system of knowledge production and transformation are the chief determinants of the romance with biology and the devaluing of social science. (Kleinman 1988:73–74)

Kleinman thus suggests, as I note in the text, that the biologization of behavior in psychotherapy is moved by interest and by a dominant system of cultural reproduction that stratifies disciplinary domains of interpretation and knowledge to position science and biology at the top of the hierarchy; biologization, he argues, is due not to the intrinsic nature of mental illness itself but to these sociocultural biases. Thus, mental health practitioners may feel both concerned and threatened by the establishment of social programs directed to address the sociocultural dimensions of mental illness; the reality of economic gain in the production, prescription, and administration of drugs pushes mental health practitioners toward the use of medication; and preventive programs do not render the same commercial benefits as this authorized (and lucrative) traffic in drugs. Furthermore, Kleinman points to the influence of the mass media, which tout research breakthroughs in the biologization of mental illness but do not dwell on the social issues that underlie its manifestations, as another factor that contributes to the reproduction of biological primacy. He argues that even the affective benefits that biologization renders for patients' families—who are thus relieved from the feelings of guilt that the presence of mental illness generates—constitute an additional circumstance that contributes to the biologization of mental illness (1988:73–74).

3. This is, of course, not unlike similar trends in the social sciences. Anthropology itself remains divided by the hard/soft dichotomy, and is located in liminal spaces that straddle the humanities and other social "sciences" which have been more "successful" in assuming the legitimating mantle of science. Within this context, as is evident from Kleinman's critique, quoted at length in the preceding note, the turn to the biologization of mental conditions and their increasing treatment through psychotropic medication is favorably viewed since it contributes to "hardening" up psychiatry, bolstering its standing among the medical sciences. Psychology likewise favors this trend. I found it significant that, at the time when I worked in the programs, clinical psychologists were lobbying for legislation that would allow them to prescribe psychotropic medication as psychiatrists and medical doctors do.

References

Acosta-Belén, Edna, and Barbara R. Sjostrom (eds.). 1988. *The Hispanic Experience in the United States*. New York: Praeger.

Aguilar, John L. 1981. "Insider Research: An Ethnography of a Debate." In D. Messerschmidt (ed.), *Anthropologists at Home in North America*, pp. 15–26. Cambridge: Cambridge University Press.

Amastae, Jon, and Lucía Elías-Olivares (eds.). 1982. *Spanish in the United States: Sociolinguistic Aspects*. Cambridge: Cambridge University Press.

American Psychiatric Association (APA). 1987. *Diagnostic and Statistical Manual of Mental Disorders* (Third Edition—Revised). Washington, D.C.: American Psychiatric Association.

———. 1994. *Diagnostic and Statistical Manual of Mental Disorders* (Fourth Edition). Washington, D.C.: American Psychiatric Association.

Anderson, Benedict. 1991. *Imagined Communities*. Rev. ed. London: Verso.

Andrade, Sally Jones. 1978. *Chicano Health: The Case of Cristal, An Evaluation of the Zavala County Mental Health Outreach Program*. Austin: The Hogg Foundation of Mental Health and the University of Texas.

Applebome, Peter. 1991. "Epilogue to Integration Fight: Blacks Favor Own Colleges." *New York Times*, 29 May, A1, A22.

Barth, Fredrik (ed.). 1969. *Ethnic Groups and Boundaries*. Boston: Little, Brown.

Bentham, Jeremy. 1995. *The Panopticon Lectures*. London: Verso.

Blauner, Robert. 1970. "Black Culture: Myth or Reality?" In N. E. Whitten and J. S. Szwed (eds.), *Afro-American Anthropology: Contemporary Perspectives*, pp. 347–66. New York: Free Press.

Blom, Jan-Petter, and John J. Gumperz. 1972. "Social Meaning in Linguistic Structures: Code-Switching in Norway." In J. J. Gumperz and D. Hymes (eds.), *Directions in Sociolinguistics*, pp. 407–434 Oxford: Basil Blackwell.

Blu, Karen. 1979. "Race and Ethnicity: Changing Symbols of Dominance and Hierarchy in the United States." *Anthropological Quarterly* 52(2):77–85.

——. 1980. *The Lumbee Problem: The Making of an American Indian People*. Cambridge: Cambridge University Press.

Bourdieu, Pierre. 1974. "The Economics of Linguistic Exchanges." *Social Science Information* 16(6):645–58.

——. 1977. *Outline of a Theory of Practice*. Translated by Richard Nice. Cambridge: Cambridge University Press.

——. 1990. *The Logic of Practice*. Translated by Richard Nice. Stanford: Stanford University Press.

——. 1991. *Language and Symbolic Power*. Edited by John B. Thompson. Translated by Gino Raymond and Matthew Adamson. Cambridge: Harvard University Press.

Bourdieu, Pierre, and Jean-Claude Passeron. 1977. *Reproduction in Education, Society, and Culture*. Translated by Richard Nice. London: Sage Publications.

Chomsky, Noam. 1988. *Language and Problems of Knowledge: The Managua Lectures*. Cambridge: MIT Press.

Cicourel, Aaron. 1980. "Language and Medicine." In C. Ferguson and S. B. Heath, *Language in the USA*, pp. 407–29. Cambridge: Cambridge University Press.

Cohn, Carol. 1987. "Sex and Death in the Rational World of Defense Intellectuals." *Signs* 12(4): 687–718.

Comaroff, John. 1992. "Of Totemism and Ethnicity." In J. and J. Comaroff, *Ethnography and the Historical Imagination*, pp. 49–67. Boulder: Westview Press.

——. 1996. "Ethnicity, Nationalism, and the Politics of Difference in an Age of Revolution." In E. N. Wilmsen and P. McAllister (eds.), *The Politics of Difference: Ethnic Premises in a World of Power*, pp. 162–83. Chicago: University of Chicago Press.

Conrad, Peter, and R. Kern (eds.). 1986. *The Sociology of Health and Disease*. New York: St. Martin's Press.

Cook, Thomas D., and William R. Shadish, Jr. 1986. "Program Evaluation: The Wordly Science." In *Annual Review of Psychology* 37:193–242.

Costantino, Giuseppe, Robert G. Malgady, and Lloyd H. Rogler. 1985. *Cuento Therapy: Folktales as a Culturally Sensitive Psychotherapy for Puerto Rican Children*. Maplewood, N.J.: Waterfront Press.

Crèvecoeur, J. Hector St. John de. 1997. *Letters from an American Farmer*. Oxford: Oxford University Press.

Crowley, Tony. 1990. "That Obscure Object of Desire: A Science of Language." In J. E. Joseph and T. J. Taylor (eds.), *Ideologies of Language*, pp. 27–50. London: Routledge.

Cuellar, Israel, and Cervando Martínez, Jr. 1984. "The Bicultural Inpatient Psychiatric Unit for Hispanic Patients at the San Antonio State Hospital." Paper prepared for the American Psychiatric Association Annual Meeting, Los Angeles, May. Authors' manuscript.

Darder, Antonia, and Rodolfo D. Torres. 1998. "Latinos and Society: Culture, Politics, and Class." In A. Darder and R. D. Torres (eds.), *The Latino Studies Reader: Culture, Economy, and Society*, pp. 3–26. Oxford: Blackwell.

Davis, Cary, Carl Haub, and JoAnne Willette. 1988. "U.S. Hispanics: Changing the Face of America. In E. Acosta-Belén and B. Sjostrom (eds.), *The Hispanic Experience in the United States*, pp. 3–55. New York: Praeger.

de Certeau, Michel. 1984. *The Practice of Everyday Life*. Berkeley: University of California Press.

de la Garza, Rodolfo O., Louis DeSipio, F. Chris García, John García, and Ángelo Falcón. 1992. *Latino Voices: Mexican, Puerto Rican, and Cuban Perspectives on American Politics*. Boulder: Westview Press.

de León, Arnoldo. 1983. *They Called Them Greasers: Anglo Attitudes toward Mexicans in Texas, 1821–1900*. Austin: University of Texas Press.

Del Castillo, Julio C. 1970. "The Influence of Language upon Symptomatology in Foreign-Born Patients." *American Journal of Psychiatry* 127(2):242–44.

di Leonardo, Micaela. 1984. *The Varieties of Ethnic Experience: Kinship, Class, and Gender among California Italian Americans*. Ithaca: Cornell University Press.

———. 1998. *Exotics at Home: Anthropologies, Others, American Modernity*. Chicago: University of Chicago Press.

Dohrenwend, Bruce P., and Barbara S. Dohrenwend. 1969. *Social Status and Psychological Disorder: A Causal Inquiry*. New York: Wiley-Interscience.

Dolgin, Daniel L., Antonio Salazar, and Salvador Cruz. 1987. "The Hispanic Treatment Program: Principles of Effective Psychotherapy." *Journal of Contemporary Psychotherapy* 17(4):285–99.

Domínguez, Virginia R. 1986. *White by Definition: Social Classification in Creole Louisiana*. New Brunswick, N.J.: Rutgers University Press.

Durán, Richard P. (ed.). 1981. *Latino Language and Communicative Behavior*. Norwood, N.J.: ABLEX Publishing Company.

Estroff, Sue E. 1981. *Making it Crazy: An Ethnography of Psychiatric Patients in an American Community*. Berkeley: University of California Press.

Evans-Pritchard, E. E. 1962. *Social Anthropology and Other Essays*. New York: Free Press.

Fábrega, Horacio. 1996. "Cultural and Historical Foundations of Psychiatric Diagnosis." In J. E. Mezzich, A. Kleinman, H. Fábrega, and D. L. Parron (eds.), *Culture and Psychiatric Diagnosis: A DSM-IV Perspective*, pp. 3–14. Washington, D.C.: American Psychiatric Association.

Fanon, Frantz. 1967. *Black Skin, White Masks*. New York: Grove Press.

Ferguson, Charles A., and Shirley Bryce Heath (eds.). 1980. *Language in the USA*. Cambridge: Cambridge University Press.

Ferrara, Kathleen Warden. 1994. *Therapeutic Ways with Words*. Oxford Studies in Sociolinguistics. New York: Oxford University Press.

Fishman, Joshua. 1972. *Language and Nationalism: Two Integrative Essays*. Rowley, Miss.: Newbury House.

———. 1997. "Do Ethnics Have Culture? And What's So Special about New York, Anyway?" In O. García and J. Fishman (eds.), *The Multilingual Apple: Languages in New York City*, pp. 3–50. Berlin: Mouton de Gruyter.

Fishman, Joshua, Robert L. Cooper, Roxanna Ma et al. 1971. *Bilingualism in the Barrio*. Bloomington: Indiana University Press.

Flores, Juan, John Attinasi, and Pedro Pedraza, Jr. 1981. "*La carreta* Made a U-Turn: Puerto Rican Language and Culture in the United States." *Daedalus* 110(2):193–217.

Flores, Juan, and George Yúdice. 1990. "Living Borders/*Buscando América*: Languages of Latino Self-formation." *Social Text* 29:57–85.

Foucault, Michel. 1965. *Madness and Civilization: A History of Insanity in the Age of Reason*. New York: Vintage Books.

———. 1972. *The Archaeology of Knowledge and the Discourse on Language*. New York: Pantheon Books.

———. 1977. *Discipline and Punish*. New York: Vintage Books.

———. 1978. *The History of Sexuality: An Introduction*. New York: Vintage Books.

———. 1980. *Power/Knowledge: Selected Interviews and Other Writings, 1972–1977*. Edited by C. Gordon. New York: Pantheon Books.

References

Franklin, Benjamin. 1992. "The German Language in Pennsylvania." In J. Crawford (ed.), *Language Loyalties: A Source Book on the Official English Controversy*, pp. 18–19. Chicago: University of Chicago Press.

Gaines, Atwood D. 1985. "The Once- and the Twice-Born: Self and Practice among Psychiatrists and Christian Psychiatrists." In R. Hahn and A. Gaines (eds.), *Physicians of Western Medicine: Anthropological Approaches to Theory and Practice*, pp. 223–46. Dordrecht: D. Reidel.

———. 1992. "Ethnopsychiatry: The Cultural Construction of Psychiatries." In *Ethnopsychiatry: The Cultural Construction of Professional and Folk Psychiatries*, pp. 3–49. Albany: State University of New York Press.

Gal, Susan. 1988. "The Political Economy of Code Choice." In M. Heller (ed.), *Codeswitching: Anthropological and Sociolinguistic Perspectives*, pp. 245–64. Berlin: Mouton de Gruyter.

García, Ofelia. 1997. "New York Multilingualism: World Languages and Their Role in a U.S. City." In O. García and J. Fishman (eds.), *The Multilingual Apple: Languages in New York City*, pp. 3–50. Berlin: Mouton de Gruyter.

Geertz, Clifford. 1973. *The Interpretation of Cultures*. New York: Basic Books.

Gerth, H. H., and C. Wright Mills (eds.). 1946. *From Max Weber: Essays in Sociology*. New York: Oxford University Press.

Giddens, Anthony. 1979. *Central Problems in Social Theory: Action, Structure, and Contradiction in Social Analysis*. Berkeley: University of California Press.

Ginsburg, Faye. 1989. *Contested Lives: The Abortion Debate in an American Community*. Berkeley: University of California Press.

Glick-Schiller, Nina. 1992. "What's Wrong with This Picture? The Hegemonic Construction of Culture in AIDS Research in the United States." *Medical Anthropology* 6(3):237–54.

Goffman, Ervin. 1959. *The Presentation of Self in Everyday Life*. New York: Doubleday.

———. 1961. *Asylums: Essays on the Social Situation of Mental Patients and Other Inmates*. New York: Doubleday.

Good, Byron J. 1994. *Medicine, Rationality, and Experience*. New York: Cambridge University Press.

Governor's Advisory Committee for Hispanic Affairs. N.d. *New York Hispanics: A Challenging Minority*. New York State Publication.

Greenwood, Davydd, Shirley Lindenbaum, Margaret Lock, and Allan Young. 1988. "Introduction: Theme Issue in Medical Anthropology." *American Ethnologist* 15:1–3.

Grimshaw, Allen D. (ed.). 1990. *Conflict Talk: Sociolinguistic Investigations of Arguments in Conversations*. Cambridge: Cambridge University Press.

Guarnaccia, Peter, Byron J. Good, and Arthur Kleinman. 1990. "A Critical Review of Epidemiological Studies of Puerto Rican Mental Health." *American Journal of Psychiatry* 147:1449–56.

Guarnaccia, Peter, and Lloyd Rogler. 1999. "Research on Culture-Bound Syndromes: New Directions." *American Journal of Psychiatry* 156:1322–27.

Gumperz, John J. 1982. *Discourse Strategies*. Cambridge: Cambridge University Press.

Gumperz, John J., and Dell Hymes (eds.). 1972. *Directions in Sociolinguistics*. Oxford: Basil Blackwell.

Gurak, Douglas T. 1988. "New York Hispanics: An Overview." In E. Acosta-Belén and B. Sjostrom (eds.), *The Hispanic Experience in the United States*, pp. 57–78. New York: Praeger.

Gutiérrez, David. 1995. *Walls and Mirrors: Mexican Americans, Mexican Immigrants, and the Politics of Identity*. Berkeley: University of California Press.

Haberman, P. 1976. "Psychiatric Symptoms among Puerto Ricans in Puerto Rico and New York City." *Ethnicity* 3:133–44.

Hahn, Robert. 1995. *Sickness and Healing: An Anthropological Perspective*. New Haven: Yale University Press.

Hahn, Robert A., and Atwood D. Gaines. 1985. *Physicians of Western Medicine: Anthropological Approaches to Theory and Practice*. Dordrecht: D. Reidel.

Hahn, Robert A., and Arthur Kleinman. 1983. "Biomedical Practice and Anthropological Theory: Frameworks and Directions." *Annual Review of Anthropology* 12:305–33.

Harwood, Alan. 1977. *Rx: Spiritist as Needed*. New York: John Wiley and Sons.

—— (ed.). 1981. *Ethnicity and Medical Care*. Cambridge: Harvard University Press.

Heller, Monica (ed.). 1988. *Codeswitching: Anthropological and Sociolinguistic Perspectives*. Berlin: Mouton de Gruyter.

Higham, John. 1963. *Strangers in the Land: Patterns of American Nativism, 1860–1925*. New York: Atheneum.

Hollingshead, August, and Fredrick Redlich. 1958. *Social Class and Mental Illness: A Community Study*. New York: John Wiley and Sons.

Hopper, Kim. 1988. "More Than Passing Strange: Homelessness and Mental Illness in New York City." *American Ethnologist* 15:155–67.

Hymes, Dell. 1972. "Models of the Interaction of Language and Social Life." In J. J. Gumperz and D. Hymes (eds.), *Directions in Sociolinguistics*, pp. 38–71. Oxford: Basil Blackwell.

——. 1974. *Foundations in Sociolinguistics: An Ethnographic Approach*. Philadelphia: University of Pennsylvania Press.

—— (ed.). 1972. *Reinventing Anthropology*. New York: Vintage Books.

Johnson, Thomas M. 1985. "Consultation-Liaison Psychiatry: Medicine as Patient, Marginality as Practice." In R. Hahn and A. Gaines (eds.), *Physicians of Western Medicine: Anthropological Perspectives in Theory and Practice*, pp. 269–92. Dordrecht: D. Reidel.

Karno, M. 1966. "The Enigma of Ethnicity in a Psychiatric Clinic." *Archives of General Psychiatry* 20:233–38.

Kleinman, Arthur. 1985. "Preface." In R. Hahn and A. Gaines (eds.), *Physicians of Western Medicine: Anthropological Approaches to Theory and Practice*, pp. vii–ix. Dordrecht: D. Reidel.

——. 1988. *Rethinking Psychiatry: From Cultural Category to Personal Experience*. New York: Free Press.

——. 1995. *Writing at the Margin: Discourse between Anthropology and Medicine*. Berkeley: University of California Press.

Kramer, Elizabeth Jane. 1977. *The New York City Health and Hospitals Corporation: Issues, Problems, and Prospects*. Chicago: Hospital Research and Educational Trust.

Labov, William, and David Fanshel. 1977. *Therapeutic Discourse: Psychotherapy as Conversation*. Orlando, Fla.: Academic Press.

Lasalle, Ivonne, and Marvette Pérez. 1997. "'Virtually' Puerto Rican: 'Dis'locating Puerto Rican-ness and Its Privileged Sites of Production." *Radical History Review* 68:54–78.

Lave, Jean. 1988. *Cognition in Practice*. Cambridge: Cambridge University Press.

Leacock, Eleanor (ed.). 1971. *The Culture of Poverty: A Critique*. New York: Simon and Schuster.

Lessinger, Johanna. 1991. "Political and Organizational Contexts of Developing Bilingual Bicultural Psychiatric Programs." Unpublished manuscript.

Levine, Elaine S., and Amado M. Padilla. 1980. *Crossing Cultures in Therapy: Counseling for Hispanics*. Monterey, Calif.: Brooks/Cole.

Lin, Wendy. 1992. "Immigrants Face New Life, New Stresses." *New York Newsday*, 9 February:69.

Lindenbaum, Shirley, and Margaret Lock (eds.). 1993. *Knowledge, Power, and Practice: The Anthropology of Medicine and Everyday Life*. Berkeley: University of California Press.

Lutz, Catherine. 1990. "Engendered Emotion: Gender, Power, and the Rhetoric of Emotional Control in American Discourse." In C. Lutz and L. Abu-Lughod, *Language and the Politics of Emotion*, pp. 69–91. Cambridge: Cambridge University Press.

Lutz, Catherine, and Lila Abu-Lughod. 1990. *Language and the Politics of Emotion*. Cambridge: Cambridge University Press.

Malgady, Robert G., Lloyd H. Rogler, and Giuseppe Costantino. 1987. "Ethnocultural and Linguistic Bias in Mental Health Evaluation of Hispanics." *American Psychologist* 42(3):228–234.

Malinowski, Bronislav. 1944. *A Scientific Theory of Culture and Other Essays*. Chapel Hill: University of North Carolina Press.

Malzberg, Benjamin. 1965. *Mental Disease among Puerto Ricans in New York State, 1960–61*. Albany: Research Foundation for Mental Hygiene.

Marcos, Luis R. 1976. "Bilinguals in Psychotherapy: Language as an Emotional Barrier." *American Journal of Psychiatry* 30:552–560.

——. 1988. "Understanding Ethnicity in Psychotherapy with Hispanic Patients." *American Journal of Psychoanalysis* 48(1):35–42.

Marcos, Luis R., Murray Alpert, Luis Urcuyo, and M. Kesselman. 1973a. "The Effect of the Interview Language on the Evaluation of Psychopathology in Spanish-American Schizophrenia Patients." *American Journal of Psychiatry* 130:549–53.

Marcos, Luis R., Luis Urcuyo, M. Kesselman, and Murray Alpert. 1973b. "The Language Barrier in Evaluating Spanish-American Patients." *Archives of General Psychiatry* 29:655–59.

Margolis, Joseph. 1976. "The Concept of Disease." *Journal of Medicine and Philosophy* 3:238–55.

Marsella, Anthony J., and Geoffrey M. White (eds.). 1982. *Cultural Conceptions of Mental Health and Therapy*. Dordrecht: D. Reidel.

Mehan, Hugh. 1990. "Oracular Reasoning in a Psychiatric Exam: The Resolution of Conflict in Language." In A. Grimshaw (ed.), *Conflict Talk: Sociolinguistic Investigations of Arguments in Conversations*, pp. 160–77. Cambridge: Cambridge University Press.

Merry, Sally Engle. 1990. *Getting Justice and Getting Even: Legal Consciousness among Working-Class Americans*. Chicago: University of Chicago Press.

Messerschmidt, Daniel (ed.). 1981. *Anthropologists at Home in North America*. Cambridge: Cambridge University Press.

Mezzich, Juan, Arthur Kleinman, Horacio Fábrega, and Dolores Parron (eds.). 1996. *Culture and Psychiatric Diagnosis: A DSM-IV Perspective*. Washington, D.C.: American Psychiatric Association.

Mollenkopf, John H. 1993. *New York City in the 1980s: A Social, Economic, and Political Atlas*. New York: Simon and Schuster.

Myers, Fred. 1988. "Locating Ethnographic Practice: Romance, Reality, and Politics in the Outback." *American Ethnologist* 15(4):609–24.

Myers, Jerome, and Lee L. Bean. 1968. *A Decade Later: A Follow-up of Social Class and Mental Illness*. New York: John Wiley and Sons.

Nader, Laura. 1972. "Up the Anthropologist: Perspectives Gained from Studying Up." In D. Hymes (ed.), *Reinventing Anthropology*, pp. 284–311. New York: Vintage Books.

Nash, June C. 1989. *From Tank Town to High Tech: The Clash of Community and Industrial Cycles*. Albany: State University of New York Press.

New York City Department of City Planning. 1990. *Comparative 1980–1990 Population and Housing Data*. New York: Population Division.

New York Times. 1992. "Census Adviser Says Poor Undercounted." 13 May:A5.

Oboler, Suzanne. 1995. *Ethnic Labels, Latino Lives: Identity and the Politics of (Re)Presentation in the United States*. Minneapolis: University of Minnesota Press.

Ochs, Elinor. 1988. *Culture and Language Development: Language Acquisition and Language Socialization in a Samoan Village*. New York: Cambridge University Press.

Ochs, Elinor, and B. B. Schieffelin. 1984. "Three Developmental Stories and Their Implications." In R. Shweder and R. A. LeVine (eds.), *Culture Theory: Essays on Mind, Self, and Emotion*, pp. 274–320. New York: Cambridge University Press.

Omi, Michael, and Howard Winant. 1994. *Racial Formation in the United States from the 1960s to the 1990s*. New York: Routledge.

Ong, Aihwa. 1987. *Spirits of Resistance and Capitalist Discipline: Factory Women in Malaysia*. Albany State University of New York Press.

Ottenberg, Simon. 1990. "Thirty Years of Fieldnotes: Changing Relationships to the Text." In R. Sanjek (ed.), *Fieldnotes: The Makings of Anthropology*, pp. 139–60. Ithaca: Cornell University Press.

Padilla, Amado, and René Ruíz. 1973. *Latino Mental Health: A Review of the Literature*. Department of Health, Education and Welfare Publications. Washington, D.C.: U.S. Government Printing Office.

Padilla, Félix. 1985. *Latino Ethnic Consciousness: The Case of Mexican Americans and Puerto Ricans in Chicago*. Notre Dame: University of Notre Dame Press.

Petersen, Alan, and Robin Bunton (eds.). 1997. *Foucault, Health, and Medicine*. London: Routledge.

Poplack, Shana. 1981. "Syntactic Structure and Social Function of Codeswitching." In R. Durán (ed.), *Latino Language and Communicative Behavior*, pp. 169–84. Norwood, N.J.: ABLEX Publishing Company.

——. 1982. "Sometimes I'll Start a Sentence in Spanish *y termino en español*: Toward a Typology of Codeswitching." In J. Amastae and L. Elías-Olivares (eds.), *Spanish in the United States: Sociolinguistic Aspects*, pp. 230–63. Cambridge: Cambridge University Press.

Price, Charles, and Israel Cuellar. 1981. "Effects of Language and Related Variables on the Expression of Psychopathology in Mexican Americans." *Hispanic Journal of Behavioral Sciences* 3:145–60.

Ramírez, Arnulfo G. 1988. "Spanish in the United States." In E. Acosta-Belén and B. Sjostrom (eds.), *The Hispanic Experience in the United States*, pp. 187–206. New York: Praeger.

Reyes, José, and Jaime Inclán. 1991. *A Study of the Mental Health Treatment of the Puerto Rican Migrant*. Monograph 1. New York: Minority Education, Research, and Training Institute.

References

Rodríguez, Clara. 1991. *Puerto Ricans Born in the USA*. Boulder: Westview Press.

Rodríguez, Clara, and Virginia Sánchez-Korrol (eds.). 1996. *Historical Perspectives on Puerto Rican Survival in the United States*. Princeton: Markus Wiener Publishers.

Romanucci-Ross, Lola, Daniel E. Moerman, and Laurence R. Tancredi. 1991. *The Anthropology of Medicine: From Culture to Method*. New York: Bergin and Garvey.

Rosado, Jaime W. 1980. "Important Psychocultural Factors in the Delivery of Mental Health Services to Lower-Class Puerto Rican Clients: A Review of Recent Studies." *Journal of Community Psychology* 8:215–26.

Ruiz, Pedro, and John Langrod. 1984. "Psychiatry and Folk Healing: A Dichotomy?" In J. E. Mezzich and C. E. Berganza (eds.), *Culture and Psychopathology*, pp. 470–75. New York: Columbia University Press.

Rushdie, Salman. 1987. *The Jaguar's Smile: A Nicaraguan Journey*. New York: Viking.

Sánchez, Rosaura. 1983 [1994]. *Chicano Discourse: Socio-Historic Perspectives*. Houston: Arte Público Press.

Sánchez-Korrol, Virginia. 1983. *From Colonia to Community: The History of Puerto Ricans in New York City*. Berkeley: University of California Press.

Sanjek, Roger (ed.). 1990. *Fieldnotes: The Makings of Anthropology*. Ithaca: Cornell University Press.

Santiago-Irizarry, Vilma. 1996. "Culture as Cure." *Cultural Anthropology* 11(1):3–24.

Sapir, Edward. 1949. "Cultural Anthropology and Psychiatry." In D. Mandelbaum (ed.), *Edward Sapir: Selected Writings in Language, Culture, and Personality*, pp. 509–21. Berkeley: University of California Press.

Schieffelin, Bambi B. 1990. *The Give and Take of Everyday Life: Language Socialization of Kaluli Children*. New York: Cambridge University Press.

Shweder, Richard, and R. LeVine. 1984. *Culture Theory: Essays on Mind, Self, and Emotion*. New York: Cambridge University Press.

Silva-Corvalán, Carmen. 1994. *Language Contact and Change: Spanish in L.A.* Oxford: Clarendon Press.

Silverstein, Michael. 1987. "Monoglot 'Standard' in America: Standardization and Metaphors of Hegemony." In R. J. Parmentier and G. Urban (eds., with the assistance of K. Pucci), *Working Papers and Proceedings of the Center for Psychosocial Studies*. Chicago: Center for Psychosocial Studies.

Silverstein, Michael, and Greg Urban (eds.). 1996. *Natural Histories of Discourse*. Chicago: University of Chicago Press.

Sollors, Werner. 1986. *Beyond Ethnicity: Consent and Descent in American Culture*. New York: Oxford University Press.

——. 1996. *Theories of Ethnicity: A Classical Reader*. New York: New York University Press.

Special Populations Sub-Task Panel on Mental Health of Hispanic Americans. 1978. *Report to the President's Commission on Mental Health*. Washington, D.C.: U.S. Government Printing Office.

Stack, Carol. 1974. *All Our Kin: Strategies for Survival in a Black Community*. New York: Harper and Row.

Starr, June, and Jane F. Collier (eds.). 1989. *History and Power in the Study of the Law: New Directions in Legal Anthropology*. Ithaca: Cornell University Press.

Steinberg, Stephen. 1989. *The Ethnic Myth: Race, Ethnicity, and Class in America*. Boston: Beacon Press.

Sue, Stanley. 1988. "Psychotherapeutic Services for Ethnic Minorities: Two Decades of Research and Findings." *American Psychologist* 43(4):301–8.

Takaki, Ronald. 1990. *Iron Cages: Race and Culture in Nineteenth-Century America*. New York: Oxford University Press.

Tambiah, Stanley. 1996. "The Nation-State in Crisis and the Rise of Ethnonationalism." In E. N. Wilmsen and P. McAllister (eds.), *The Politics of Difference: Ethnic Premises in a World of Power*, pp. 124–43. Chicago: University of Chicago Press.

Taussig, Michael. 1980. "Reification and the Consciousness of the Patient." *Social Science and Medicine* 14:3–13.

Thompson, John B. 1991. "Editor's Introduction." In P. Bourdieu, *Language and Symbolic Power*, pp. 1–31. Translated by Gino Raymond and Matthew Adamson. Cambridge: Harvard University Press.

Torres, Lourdes. 1997. *Puerto Rican Discourse: A Sociolinguistic Study of a New York City Suburb*. Mahwah, N.J.: Lawrence Erlbaum Associates.

Turner, Bryan S. 1984. *The Body and Society: Explorations in Social Theory*. Oxford: Basil Blackwell.

Urciuoli, Bonnie. 1991. "The Political Topography of Spanish and English: The View from a New York Puerto Rican Neighborhood." *American Ethnologist* 18(2):295–310.

——. 1996. *Exposing Prejudice: Puerto Rican Experiences of Language, Race, and Class*. Boulder: Westview Press.

Valentine, Charles A. 1968. *Culture and Poverty: Critiques and Counterproposals*. Chicago: University of Chicago Press.

Weber, Max. 1946. "Science as a Vocation." In H. H. Gerth and C. W. Mills (eds.), *From Max Weber: Essays in Sociology*, pp. 129–56. New York: Oxford University Press.

Whorf, Benjamin. 1956. "The Relation of Habitual Thought and Behavior to Language." In J. B. Carroll (ed.), *Language, Thought, and Reality: Selected Writings of Benjamin Lee Whorf*, pp. 134–59. Cambridge: MIT Press.

Williams, Brackette. 1989. "A Class Act: Anthropology and the Race to Nation across Ethnic Terrain." *Annual Review of Anthropology* 18:401–44.

——. 1991. *Stains on my Name, War in my Veins: Guyana and the Politics of Cultural Struggle*. Durham: Duke University Press.

Wilmsen, Edwin N. 1996. "Introduction: Premises of Power in Ethnic Politics." In E. N. Wilmsen and P. McAllister, *The Politics of Difference: Ethnic Premises in a World of Power*, pp. 1–24. Chicago: University of Chicago Press.

Woolard, Kathryn. 1989. *Double Talk: Bilingualism and the Politics of Ethnicity in Catalonia*. Stanford: Stanford University Press.

Young, Allan. 1982. "The Anthropologies of Illness and Sickness." *Annual Review of Anthropology* 11:257–85.

Zentella, Ana Celia. 1980. "Language Variety among Puerto Ricans." In C. A. Ferguson and S. B. Heath (eds.), *Language in the U.S.*, pp. 218–39. Cambridge University Press.

——. 1981. "'Tá bien, You Could Answer Me *en cualquier idioma*." In R. Durán (ed.), *Latino Language and Communicative Behavior*, pp. 169–84. Norwood, N.J.: ABLEX Publishing Company.

——. 1982. "Codeswitching and Interactions among Puerto Rican Children." In J. Amastae and L. Elías-Olivares (eds.), *Spanish in the United States: Sociolinguistic Aspects*, pp. 230–63. Cambridge: Cambridge University Press.

References

——. 1990a. "Integrating Qualitative and Quantitative Methods in the Study of Bilingual Code Switching." In *The Uses of Linguistics*, pp. 75–92. New York: Annals of the New York Academy of Sciences.

——. 1990b. "Return Migration, Language and Identity: Puerto Rican Bilinguals in *dos* Worlds/Two *mundos.*" *International Journal of Society and Language* 84:81–100.

——. 1997. *Growing Up Bilingual: Puerto Rican Children in New York City*. London: Blackwell.

Zola, Irving K. 1986. "Medicine as an Institution of Social Control." In P. Conrad and R. Kern (eds.), *The Sociology of Health and Disease*, pp. 379–94. New York: St. Martin's Press.

Index

African Americans: as administrators, 74–75, 79; attitude of, toward Latino programs, 49, 51; and mental health issues, 102–104; ward for, 78. *See also* Bilingual, bicultural psychiatric programs; Cultural sensitivity; Discourse; Essentializing; Ethnicity; Latinos; Negotiations; Politics of identity; Race

Ambiance: components of, 60–62, 80–82; as cultural reification, 85–87; and cultural sensitivity, 18, 57; as embodiment of Latino values, 106; in evaluation design, 17; and milieu therapy, 59–60, 63; in program proposal, 16, 55; as strategy, 80–82, 85. *See also* Cultural sensitivity; Mental illness

Anthropology, 5; in evaluation project, 57, 77; and exoticism, 6, 154n. 4; and psychiatry, 33; of the United States, 11–12, 130, 154n. 4. *See also* Medical anthropology; Methodology; Reflexivity

Bilingual, bicultural psychiatric programs, 14–15, 47–53, 147; competition among, 20; and evaluation design, 17–18; goals of, 16–17; ideology and, 20; evaluation proposal for, 53–55; staffing of, 119–121, 157n. 3, 161–162nn. 3, 4; therapeutic group activities in, 128–139. *See also* Latino mental health practitioners; Mental health institutions; Mental illness; Policy-making; *individual programs*

Closed institutions. *See* Total or closed institutions

Contrastive strategies, 21, 26, 80, 148. *See also* Essentializing; Ethnicity; Politics of identity; Primordialism; Race

Cultural sensitivity, 15–18; and African Americans, 103; and "folk" religions, 117–118; and institutions, 5; Latino definitions of, 18–19; and medicine, 1–2, 145; and milieu therapy, 60; and otherness, 104; and paraprofessional staff, 122–123; and policy-making, 5; in programs' design, 55; in research center, 22; as strategy, 140; training in, 61–62. *See also* Ambiance; Culture; Language; Latino mental health practitioners; Politics of identity

Culture: as "content," 22, 87, 143–144; as knowledge, 108, 113; and language, 51–52; and medicine, 3, 147; pathologized, 69, 112–113; and policy-making, 6; and psychiatry, 5, 16–17, 33, 41–42, 100, 136–139, 149–150, 154–155n. 3, 160n. 7; reified, 43, 57, 62, 82–85, 146; as strategy, 16, 20–22. *See also* Cultural sensitivity; Discourse; Essentializing; Ideology; Language; Primordialism

"Culture of poverty," 40–43

Discourse: on cultural sensitivity, 18–19, 55; on culture, 5; definition of, 4, 153n. 1; of entitlement, 43, 46–47, 77; on identity, 113–114, 123–126, 139; of labor rights, 64; on language, 106–112; on "Latinization," 92–94; on race and ethnicity, 24–29; racializing and ethnicizing, 27–28; as strategy, 5, 53; as "translation," 140–143. *See also* Language; Practices

Essentializing: and ambiance, 80, 85–87; and the census, 90; and institutions, 4–5; and policy-making, 5; in race and ethnicity, 28; of researchers, 3, 30; as strategy, 5, 21, 94, 110, 113–119. *See also* Culture; Ethnicity; Ideology; Primordialism; Race; Reflexivity

Ethnic activism, 7; and the census, 91–95; Latino organization and, 45–46, 48–55; in mental health, 39; and self-interest, 14. *See also* Evaluation; Latino mental health practitioners; Latinos; Negotiations; Numbers argument

Ethnic consciousness: definition of, 22, 155n. 7; practical and discursive, 26

Ethnicity: as cognition, 22; as "content," 3, 22; definition of, 5; and medicalization, 1–8; and policy-making, 38; and race, 24–29, 155–156nn. 8, 9; as strategy, 82–85, 87; in the United States, 12, 25, 156n. 4. *See also* Culture; Essentializing; Ideology; Language; Latinos; Primordialism; Race; Reflexivity

"Ethnicization" of mental health, 2, 18–19; and bilingual, bicultural psychiatric programs, 13

Evaluation: anthropological methods in, 22; design of, 17, 22, 29; ideology and, 19; political nature of, 19, 29; process of, 19–20; in programs' goals, 17–18; project of, 13, 52; proposal for, 53; and research center, 55–57. *See also* Ethnic activism; Methodology; Negotiations; Reflexivity

Governor's Committee for Hispanic Affairs, New York State, 50

Habitus: definition of, 154n. 2; among mental health practitioners, 17

Health and Hospitals Corporation (HHC), New York City, 47, 74

Hispanics. *See* Latinos

Ideology: of bilingual, bicultural psychiatric programs, 54–55, 67, 80–82; of capitalist redistribution, 91–92; and the census, 90; of identity, 24, 38, 91, 146–147; institutional, 48–53, 59–60; of language, 89, 96–98, 106–112; in policy-making, 43; psychiatric, 18, 33, 46, 89, 117–118, 126–128, 134–135; in scientific framework, 17–18; in the United States, 3–5, 11, 147. *See also* Culture; Discourse; Essentializing; Ethnicity; Institutions; Language; Latino mental health practitioners; Medicalization; Multiculturalism; Practices; Primordialism; Psychiatry; Race

Institutions: closed or total, 58–59; definition of, 153n. 1; and evaluation, 29; politics of, 37–38, 47–53, 63; practices of, 5; processes of, 5, 16, 25. *See also* Bilingual, bicultural psychiatric programs; Cultural sensitivity; Essentializing; Evaluation; Ideology; Latino mental health practitioners; Medicalization; Mental health institutions; Practices; Primordialism

Jefferson Hospital, 14; history of, 74–76; organization of, 75–76, 78–80; patient population of, 76–77; physical description of, 74–76, 77–78; staff of, 75. *See also* Bilingual, bicultural psychiatric programs; Ethnic activism; Evaluation; Latino mental health practitioners; Negotiations

Language: and ambiance, 81, 85; as barrier, 39–44, 46, 48; and culture, 87, 153n. 1, 155n. 4; Latino bilingualism and, 16, 27; Latino diversity in, 23, 89, 132–133; Latino monolingualism and, 16, 21; and medicine, 4–5, 99–100; pathologized, 54, 135; and psychiatry, 4–5, 88–89, 100–102, 106–112, 160n. 7; "regression" in, 16, 54–55, 89, 95–100; as strategy, 15, 28, 51–53. *See also* Bilingual, bicultural psychiatric programs; Cultural sensitivity; Culture; Discourse; Ideology; Essentializing; Latino mental health practitioners; Latinos; Primordialism

"Latinization" of the United States, 92–94

Latino mental health practitioners: as activists, 21; and cultural sensitivity, 2, 15; as cultural and professional authorities,

Anthropology of Contemporary Issues

A SERIES EDITED BY

ROGER SANJEK

The Anthropology of Contemporary Issues

A Series Edited by

ROGER SANJEK

A full list of titles in the series appears at the end of this book.

Medicalizing Ethnicity